The Danger of Puberty Suppression

The Danger of Puberty Suppression

An Ethical Evaluation of Suppressing Puberty in
Gender-Dysphoric Children from a Christian Perspective

MICHAEL S. DELLAPERUTE

Foreword by Mark McGinniss

RESOURCE *Publications* · Eugene, Oregon

THE DANGER OF PUBERTY SUPPRESSION
An Ethical Evaluation of Suppressing Puberty in Gender-Dysphoric Children from a Christian Perspective

Resource Publications
An Imprint of Wipf and Stock Publishers
199 W. 8th Ave., Suite 3
Eugene, OR 97401

www.wipfandstock.com

PAPERBACK ISBN: 978-1-5326-8499-9
HARDCOVER ISBN: 978-1-5326-8500-2
EBOOK ISBN: 978-1-5326-8506-4

Manufactured in the U.S.A.   AUGUST 16, 2019

To my wife, Michelle, my best friend, biggest supporter, the mother of my children, and the love of my life!

Contents

Foreword

YOU ARE HOLDING THIS book in your hand or (more accurately probably) reading it electronically, because you are confused about gender dysphoria. You have come to a resource that unravels the so-called confusion and speaks truth to a heart-wrenching situation.

Gender dysphoria does not simply cause great confusion in a child; it also produces grave bewilderment for his or her parents, medical providers, and ministry professionals. With candor, compassion, and biblical wisdom, Dellaperute untangles the confusion to aid those who are responsible for our precious children. This is extremely important since in the case of gender dysphoria the proverbial cure (transition) is physically and emotionally far more dangerous than the gender confusion itself.

At present, however, the loudest voices concerning gender dysphoria are those advocating some level of transition—at any cost—even at the cost of the physical and emotional well-being of the gender-confused child. Dellaperute demonstrates scientifically that there is no known medical cause for gender dysphoria and thus radical medical intervention such as hormones and gender reassignment surgeries are medically, ethically, and biblically inappropriate to help parents or their child deal with the confusion.

Dellaperute's voice is only a small, contrary voice among the din of those who advocate radical medical intervention to deal with the subjective self-diagnosis of a gender-confused child. But his is a voice that must be heeded since the very lives and future of our children are at stake. Our children are too precious to be left to deal with this confusion in a manner that flies in the face of the way they were created by God.

With sympathetic clarity this book offers a succinct understanding of gender dysphoria for parents, medical providers, ministry professionals, and even the child. To advocate for any position or action that does not honor the divine design in each unique child is guilty of the most perverse form of child abuse.

MARK MCGINNISS, PH.D.

1

What Happens When it is Your Child?

As a parent, you fear that there is something seriously wrong with your child, and you do not know what to do.

Your concern for the health and safety of your child first surfaced as they began to approach puberty. You watched a once happy and well-adjusted child grow increasingly anxious, despondent, and isolated with each passing season.[1] In spite of your best efforts, your child flatly refused to participate in any gender-typical activities. Over time, you even discovered a cache of gender-atypical toys and clothing hidden in their room.[2] When you finally confronted your child about their gender-nonconforming behaviors, they confessed a belief that their true inner self was not congruent with their natal gender. In short, they felt they were trapped in

---

1. Puckett et al., "Barriers to Gender-affirming Care," 54. Contrary to popular cultural narratives, most transgender and gender non-conforming (TGNC) individuals did not exhibit symptoms of gender dysphoria (most commonly anxiety and depression) from early childhood. One 27-year-old female-to-male transgender admits to Puckett et al. in a blind survey, "I pretended I'd always hated my body and 'always' knew I was a boy. I didn't" (54).

2. Hruz et al., "Growing Pains," 20. Hruz et al. explain that the subjective nature of a gender dysphoria diagnosis in children relies on, "Gender-atypical behaviors (for example, boys playing with dolls or girls preferring to play with boys)" (20).

the wrong body, and they wanted you to help them fix their problem by transitioning to the opposite gender. Now, you have heard about other children making these kinds of claims. You have seen them on the news or read about them online. But this is your child. So what will you do?

Let's assume you were like most parents. If so, then your initial response to your child would have included a mixture of disbelief and frustration.[3] Eventually, you even dismissed their self-assessment as a passing phase.[4] Maybe you even informed your child that they were assigned a gender at conception based on their chromosomes. It is basic biology, right? XX chromosomes mean that you are a female, and XY chromosomes mean that you are a male. As a result, you explained that gender transition was not a possibility. At best, while their body could conceivably be altered to resemble the opposite gender to some degree, this would require a long, painful, expensive, irreversible, and truly imperfect process that could never achieve gender change on the chromosomal level. That is just basic science. As a parent, you assumed your explanation would settle the matter. However, your refusal to affirm your child's gender identity only seemed to accentuate their distress. So your child took the initiative to meet with a school counselor,[5] and they become fixated with online transgender media sources.[6] Soon your elementary school-aged child began to

3. Harris, "I'd Rather Have a Living Son." TGNC children and teens report that their parents commonly responded to their coming out with disbelief or anger.

4. Singal, "Your Child Says She's Trans," 90. The self-diagnosis of gender dysphoria in children and teens is a major factor in gender-affirming care.

5. Calfas, "An Ohio Bill." In some states like Ohio, there is at present an intense legal battle being waged between LGBT advocates and parents over the issue of parental consent. Ohio lawmakers believe it is the parents' right to consent to any treatment offered to their child. LGBT activists argue that TGNC children should be treated autonomously, without parental consent. Like other cultural issues, this argument is gaining traction in several states.

6. Singal, "Your Child Says She's Trans," 90. Not by coincidence, media influence has a profound impact on TGNC children and teens. Concerning the struggles of a 14-year-old female named "Claire," Signal reports, "Claire started watching YouTube videos made by young people. She was particularly

drop terms like "transphobic," "gender dysphoria," "discriminatory," and, of course, "puberty suppressors."

Within months, your child steadily grew more vocal about their convictions, insisting that family members, teachers, and classmates alike refer to them by a different name associated with their expressed gender. Your child also grew increasingly belligerent toward anyone who refused to support their decision uncritically. The conflict in your home finally came to a head when your child insisted on cross-dressing for a public function. Your refusal to support their behavior resulted in a heated argument. After allowing time for your child's anger to subside, you entered their room only to find them huddled in a corner, sobbing, and cutting their arm with the sharp edge of a paper clip.[7] That was the moment you wrapped your arms around your child and promised to get them help. But silently you wondered, "What does help look like? What is the right response to this situation? After all, they are still just a child. Should I pursue the kind of help that will ultimately alter their body so that it better aligns with their mind? Or should I seek the kind of help that focuses on correcting their thinking so that it more accurately aligns with their body? And, are these my only options?"

Later that evening you log on to an online forum that promises to provide answers for confused parents of Transgender and Gender Non-conforming (TGNC) children. In desperation, you describe your child's condition to strangers on the internet. The reply comes within minutes: "If your child says they are trans, then they are trans. If your child says they need hormones, then it is your responsibility to help get them on hormones. The most

---

fascinated by . . . Miles McKenna, a charismatic 22-year-old. His 1 million subscribers have followed along as he came out as a trans boy, went on testosterone, got a double mastectomy, and transformed into a happy, healthy young man. Claire had discovered the videos by accident, or rather by algorithm: They showed up in her 'recommended' stream. They gave a name to Claire's discomfort. She began to wonder whether she was transgender" (90).

7. Harris, "I'd Rather Have a Living Son." TGNC children and teens such as "Martin" often report cutting or other acts of self-mutilation.

important thing you can do is affirm your child."[8] When you question whether or not this is an appropriate course of action, the online experts quickly respond, "Would you rather have a dead son or a live daughter?"[9] So here you stand, convinced that there is something seriously wrong with your child, but unsure about what steps to take next. How will you address a moral conflict that will affect your child for the rest of their life? Where will you turn to find help? Is this truly a case where choosing the lesser evil provides a satisfactory ethical solution to your moral dilemma?[10]

Hold that thought, and let's consider this same situation from another angle. Instead of the parent, now you are the doctor or medical care provider.

A parent and their prepubescent child are waiting for you in the examination room. When you arrive, the parent assumes the role of advocate and proceeds to do most of the talking before you have a chance to assess your young patient. The parent informs you that their child is gender dysphoric. It is clear, both from the description they give and the terminology they implement, that they have done significant research on this subject and have already initiated social transition with their child. When finally questioned, the child confirms their parent's narrative. The child insists that the anatomical features associated with their natal gender cause them significant emotional distress. They also identify an array of supporting symptoms that include anxiety, depression, and suicidal thoughts. The child appears convinced that the only

8. Singal, "Your Child Says She's Trans," 90. This is a paraphrase of the actual advice that "Heather," the mother of "Claire," received when she was searching for help for her TGNC daughter online.

9. Harris, "I'd Rather Have a Living Son." This popular defeater is often employed as an appeal to nonaffirming parents. It was used by Erica Kasper as moral justification for her support of the gender transition of her FtM TGNC teenager in a documentary aired on WNYC radio.

10. Geisler, *Christian Ethics*, 98. Geisler explains that conflicting absolutism acknowledges a moral conflict and elects to choose the lesser of two evils. In the case of a parent reluctant to accept their TGNC child, the appeal to conflicting absolutism places more weight on the life of the child than on the gender identity of the child, thereby allowing moral justification for gender transition. The thesis of this book will proceed to challenge this approach.

solution to their problem is gender transition, and they express persistent dread over the onset of puberty.

At this point in the dialogue, the parent is distraught. They insist it is medically necessary to take every measure to protect their child from any self-destructive tendencies.[11] They explain that these measures include the immediate prescription of puberty-suppressing hormones.[12] The parent then presents you with written recommendations and printed testimonials they received after their child's first meeting with a professional gender-affirming therapist.[13] These testimonials describe puberty suppression as a safe, reliable, tested, and fully reversible treatment plan for children with gender dysphoria.[14]

Years of training cause you to hesitate before writing the prescription. You begin by explaining to both parties that, in your professional medical opinion, the child not only lacks the necessary competency to make a decision of this magnitude, but they have not been comprehensively examined. Furthermore, prescribing the requested drugs may result in serious consequences that the child will later regret if their distress desists.[15] By the time you are finished, the parent is irate. They respond to your explanations with accusations of gatekeeping and discrimination.[16] They de-

---

11. Puckett et al., "Barriers to Gender-affirming Care," 53. Puckett et al. use their survey results to argue that it is necessity to provide pharmaceutical and medical means to TGNC individuals.

12. Puckett et al., "Barriers to Gender-affirming Care," 54. Puckett et al. state that TGNC individuals seeking medical intervention felt like they needed to, "Educate their providers," believed they regularly encountered bias, and, "Felt that the guidelines suggesting that they obtain letters from therapists were problematic" (54).

13. Singal, "Your Child Says She's Trans," 92. Even though there is no objective medical standard used to diagnose gender dysphoria, Singal documents that professional therapists have, "After a 20-minute evaluation, pronounced the child trans" (92).

14. Coleman et al., "Standards of Care," 18. This source will be referred to as WPATH's *Standards of Care*. WPATH's *Standards of Care* maintains that the effects of synthetic puberty-suppressing hormones are "Fully reversible" (18).

15. Coleman et al., "Standards of Care," 11.

16. Puckett et al., "Barriers to Gender-affirming Care," 53–54.

mand treatment, and threaten you with legal action if you refuse. So what will you do? Will you act against your professional integrity and regard the self-diagnosis of a pre-pubescent patient and untrained parent as though it were authoritative?[17] Or will you potentially place both your patient's life and your medical practice at risk by conscientiously refusing to treat the child with puberty suppressors?[18] Ethically, do you even have a choice in the matter? What is the right response to this complicated and emotionally charged situation?

Before we explore the answer to that question, keep in mind that the impact of puberty-suppressing hormones does not end at the home or doctor's office. So let's consider one final scenario. Instead of the parent or the doctor, let's assume that you are now the ministry professional.

A family in your church has requested a meeting with you in order to discuss their concerns regarding the treatment of their child. During the appointment, they disclose that their child has been diagnosed with gender dysphoria. This diagnosis, initiated by the child, was affirmed by a professional counselor. The parents intend to follow the counselor's recommendation and allow gender transition to proceed at the child's discretion.[19] Furthermore, a medical professional has recently prescribed drugs that will suppress the onset of puberty, ultimately allowing for smoother transition. The family requests that the church adopt a policy of acceptance toward the child's decision to explore their gender identity and transition fully at a later date. This policy would include allowing the child to use the restroom of their expressed gender, calling the child by their newly chosen name and preferred pronouns, affirming the child's choice of clothing and activities, and supporting the family through the transition process, beginning with the suppression of puberty.

17. Beauchamp and Childress, *Principles of Biomedical Ethics*, 41.

18. Beauchamp and Childress, *Principles of Biomedical Ethics*, 43.

19. Dellaperute, "Church and the Transgender Issue," 90. See my article for a detailed explanation of social, chemical, and physical transition.

The parents believe that a gender affirmation method of treatment for gender dysphoria is in the best interest of the child. However, when you question whether this is the right course of action due to your biblical convictions of a fixed male and female gender binary based on the creation narrative in Scripture,[20] you are met with a harsh reaction. Both parents warn you that, if the church will not affirm their child's gender identity, they will have no choice but to break fellowship and possibly pursue legal recourse for emotional and spiritual abuse. They wonder aloud, "How can a loving church choose to ignore such a simple request to help a child?" You wonder, "How do I respond to this situation in an ethical manner? Does the Bible offer moral guidance for addressing the issue of gender, parenting, or the suppression of puberty?"

If you, as a parent, medical provider, or ministry professional, think these situations will never happen to you, then you need to think again. They are occurring at an alarming rate. Jesse Singal reports, "The number of self-identifying trans people in the United States is on the rise . . . As of 2017 . . . about 150,000 teenagers ages 13 to 17 identified as trans. The number of young people seeking clinical services appears to be growing as well."[21] So, what would you do if a child in your life was advocating for puberty-suppressing hormones? Does this treatment plan, which is promoted as gender-affirming, help children or hurt them? Is it ethical, or biblical, to halt puberty for the purpose of gender transition? And what happens if the child changes their mind in the near or distant future? These are the questions that this book will help you answer.

---

20. Beauchamp and Childress, *Principles of Biomedical Ethics*, 106. Beauchamp and Childress explain that shared ethical norms with religious institutions do not prevent these norms from being autonomously accepted.

21. Singal, "Your Child Says She's Trans," 91.

2

How Do You Speak the New Language of Gender?

IN ALL LIKELIHOOD, SOME of the terms from the previous chapter, like "natal gender" or "gender dysphoria," were unfamiliar to you, since most of them are relatively new. The first step to helping a child navigate the treacherous terrain of contemporary gender dysphoria and TGNC treatment plans is to gain a basic understanding of the new language of gender. Postmodern deconstructionism plays a prominent role in the current transgender terminology employed by proponents of gender affirmation. "Gender affirmation" is an umbrella term for the course of treatment that advocates for the use of puberty-suppressing hormones in gender-dysphoric children. As a result, new vocabulary is regularly being developed by gender affirmation activists, while existing terms are either being redefined or reclassified as offensive or discriminatory at an astounding rate, creating an ever-changing dynamic that is rife with relativism.[1] As Singal reports, "A rich new language has taken root, granting kids who may have felt excluded the words they need to describe their experiences."[2] For example, Puckett et al. warn

---

1. Walker, *God and the Transgender Debate*, 21.
2. Singal, "Your Child Says She's Trans," 91.

medical professionals, "When directly interacting with TGNC patients, providers should avoid disrespectful language. Phrases like 'biological,' . . . should not be used."[3] Consider the implications of this assessment: Gender experts are recommending that the term "biological" be removed from the vocabulary of medical professionals because it offends individuals who reject their biological make-up. Parents, medical providers, and ministry professionals need to learn to how to speak this new language of gender.

When attempting to engage a culture where physicians are advised against referring to biology at the risk of being perceived as disrespectful, it is essential to define pertinent contemporary terminology before proceeding to evaluate treatment methods of gender-dysphoric and TGNC children, beginning with natal gender. "Natal gender" is the current term that has replaced "biological gender," "birth gender," or "the assigned sex of an individual."[4] The delivery-room exclamations, "It's a boy," or "It's a girl,"[5] are examples of natal gender.[6] The natal gender of gender-dysphoric and TGNC individuals differs from their expressed/experienced gender. "Experienced gender" describes the subjective or fluid gender expression of an individual often associated with social transition.[7] "I am a boy who prefers to dress and act like a girl," is an example of expressed gender. These gender expressions are broad enough to include boys in blue shirts with buzz cuts and girls in pink dresses with pony tails. Gender expression differs slightly from

3. Puckett et al., "Barriers to Gender-affirming Care," 57. Whether or not a doctor should be permitted to appeal to biological factors when assessing a patient without being labeled as biased is beyond the scope of this book. However, it is telling to note that the descriptive term "biological" has been labeled "disrespectful" to TGNC patients.

4. Many of the sources cited in this work, while published within the last decade, predate the latest fluid terminology. As a result, some sources will refer to outdated terms such as "biological gender" or "GID."

5. Compton, "'Boy or girl?'" A developing cultural trend is to raise genderless children, recently dubbed, "Theybies."

6. Walker, *God and the Transgender Debate*, 29–30. Walker identifies the ironic nature of a society that celebrates gender-reveal parties for pregnant women while facilitating gender transition for children.

7. Hruz et al., "Growing Pains," 3–4.

gender identity. WPATH's *Standards of Care*, 7th Edition, the most recent edition provided by the most vocal supporters of gender affirmation at the time of this printing, defines gender identity as, "A person's intrinsic sense of being male (a boy or man) or female (a girl or woman), or an alternative gender."[8] For example, a child may state, "Regardless of my natal gender, I identify as a girl." In contrast to the objective nature of natal gender, gender identity is commonly perceived to be subjective.[9] Furthermore, gender identity is typically divided into two the categories of cisgender and gender nonconforming (GNC).

"Cisgender" describes individuals whose gender identity and expression aligns with their natal gender. A cisgender natal female may declare, "I am a girl who likes to wear pink dresses and play with dolls." GNC, sometimes referred to as gender variant (GV), genderqueer, or gender diverse in the ever-changing linguistic landscape,[10] refers to an individual whose gender identity or expression does not align with social norms. A GNC natal male may state, "I am a boy who likes to wear pink dresses and play with dolls." To further complicate the issue, advocates of gender affirmation such as Meier and Harris observe that the GNC child may transcend the bounds of binary gender, effectively declaring, "I'm a boy on the bottom and a girl on the top."[11] This terminology reflects a growing trend in popular culture to reject the gender binary of male and female as defined in Scripture (Gen 1:26–27) in favor of a more diverse, culturally constructed gender spectrum. A persistent GNC child may ultimately be classified as gender dysphoric, a condition formerly known as gender identity disorder (GID).

Coleman et al. define gender dysphoria (GD) in WPATH's *Standards of Care* as, "Distress that is caused by a discrepancy between a person's gender identity and that person's assigned sex

---

8. Coleman et al., "Standards of Care," 96.

9. Firth, "Childhood Abuse and Depressive Vulnerability," 298.

10. Meier and Harris, "Fact Sheet."

11. Meier and Harris, "Fact Sheet," para. 1.

at birth."[12] WPATH is an acronym for the World Professional Association for Transgender Health, a leading nonprofit gender affirmation organization whose website states that they are:

> Devoted to transgender health. Our professional, supporting, and student members engage in clinical and academic research to develop evidence-based medicine and strive to promote a high quality of care for transsexual, transgender, and gender-nonconforming individuals.[13]

According to WPATH's *Standards of Care,* the presence of distress marks the difference between GNC and gender dysphoria.[14] For example, a gender-dysphoric natal male may explain, "I hate being a boy who likes to wear pink dresses and play with dolls. I want to be a girl." However, WPATH's definition of gender dysphoria is far from exhaustive. Dr. Michele Cretella, president of the American College of Pediatricians and critic of WPATH's gender affirmation approach, further explains that gender dysphoria is, "A psychological condition in which they experience marked incongruence between their experienced gender and the gender associated with their biological sex."[15] Ristori and Steensma expound upon the most current set of distressing factors that contribute to a diagnosis of gender dysphoria in childhood, stating:

> According to the DSM–5, a diagnosis of GD of childhood can be made if a child experiences a marked incongruence between one's experienced/expressed gender and assigned gender, of at least 6 months' duration, as manifested by six out of eight criteria. One *sine qua non* criterion must be the experience of a strong desire to be of another gender or an insistence to be another gender. In addition to this, there are two criteria focusing on anatomic dysphoria; a dislike of one's sexual anatomy and the desire for primary/secondary sex characteristics of the experienced gender. In addition there are five

12. Coleman et al., "Standards of Care," 96.
13. https://www.wpath.org/about/mission-and-vision, para. 1.
14. Coleman et al., "Standards of Care," 5.
15. Cretella, "Gender Dysphoria in Children," 287.

behavioural [*sic*] criteria. The behavioural criteria concern the preference for cross-dressing; adopting cross-gender roles in fantasy play; a strong preference for toys, games and activities of the other gender; a preference for playmates of the other gender; and a strong aversion or rejection of typically gender congruent roles, interests, preferences and behaviours. Furthermore, the condition is associated with clinically significant distress or impairment in social, school, or other important areas of functioning.[16]

In an earlier ethical evaluation of hormone treatment, Brendan Abel claims, "Gender dysphoria can be diagnosed in childhood—as young as three years old."[17] According to the DSM–5 manual and WPATH standards, a prepubescent, GNC, natal female who declares, "Since I identify as a boy, my natal gender causes me distress," would need to exhibit this distress consistently and persistently for a period of at least 6 months in order to qualify as gender dysphoric. These are the standards that gender affirmation advocates claim to adhere to when treating gender-dysphoric children. However, pressure from advocacy groups for immediate treatment of GNC children has led to the creation of the latest term, Rapid Onset Gender Dysphoria (ROGD). According to Lisa Littman, "Rapid-onset gender dysphoria describes a phenomenon where the development of gender dysphoria is observed to begin suddenly during or after puberty in an adolescent or young adult who would not have met criteria for gender dysphoria in childhood."[18] The new diagnosis of ROGD will likely afford gender-dysphoric adolescents swifter access to gender transition procedures, including puberty suppression.

While all transgender (T) individuals are gender dysphoric, not all individuals with gender dysphoria are automatically considered transgender. Puckett et al. define transgender as, "An umbrella term that refers to individuals who do not identify

16. Ristori and Steensma, "Gender Dysphoria in Childhood," 13.

17. Abel, "Hormone Treatment of Children," S23.

18. Littman, "Rapid-onset Gender Dysphoria," 37.

with the gender that is typically associated with someone of their sex assigned at birth."[19] Puckett's definition differs slightly from WPATH's *Standards of Care*, which defines transgender as an, "Adjective to describe a diverse group of individuals who cross or transcend culturally defined categories of gender. The gender identity of transgender people differs to varying degrees from the sex they were assigned at birth."[20] Meier and Harris capture the contemporary catchphrase for identifying transgender youth by maintaining, "Transgender children typically consistently, persistently, and insistently express a cross-gender identity and feel their gender is different from their assigned sex."[21] A transgender natal female may insist, "Since I identify and express as a male, my distress can only be resolved by transitioning to become a male." The acronym TGNC currently incorporates both transgender and gender nonconformists. The complications of gender-dysphoric and TGNC children are compounded at puberty, when the physical differences between natal males and natal females become more pronounced by the development of primary and secondary sexual characteristics.

Kuper identifies "puberty" as the term used to describe a time in life when drastic changes occur in, "Body structures, body functions, and physical appearance."[22] These changes ultimately result in adolescents reaching sexual maturity. Hruz et al., themselves critics of gender affirmation, note that while the age of puberty onset varies greatly from one individual to another, gonads typically begin to mature in natal females between the ages of eight and thirteen and in natal males between the ages of nine and fourteen.[23] Puberty-suppressing hormones, also known as puberty blockers or gonadotrophin-releasing hormone (GnRH) analogues/agonists, are administered to gender-dysphoric and TGNC children in order to prevent some of the undesired physical changes

19. Puckett et al., "Barriers to Gender-affirming Care," 48.

20. Coleman et al., "Standards of Care," 97.

21. Meier and Harris, "Fact Sheet," para. 2.

22. Kuper, "Puberty Blocking Medications," 2.

23. Hruz et al., "Growing Pains," 8.

of puberty from manifesting. These changes primarily relate to the development of primary and secondary sexual characteristics. Kuper maintains:

> Puberty blockers are a medical treatment available to support the healthy development of transgender adolescents. By halting puberty, puberty blockers have been shown to reduce gender dysphoria (e.g., discomfort with sex characteristics) and promote mental health.[24]

However, contrary to Kuper, puberty blockers do not halt puberty entirely, nor were they developed for treatment of gender-dysphoric and TGNC children, nor do they promote the healthy development of human beings. Presently, puberty suppressors remain an untested and off-label use for gender-dysphoric and TGNC adolescents. Hruz et al. clarify:

> Hormone interventions to suppress puberty were not developed for the purpose of treating children with gender dysphoria—rather, they were first used as a way to normalize puberty for children who undergo puberty too early, a condition known as "precocious puberty." For females, precocious puberty is defined as the onset of puberty before age 8, while for males it is defined as the onset of puberty before age 9.[25]

Proponents of the gender affirmation approach to treating gender dysphoria favor the administration of puberty-suppressing hormones to gender-dysphoric and TGNC children for two primary reasons. First, Giovanardi explains that proponents of the gender affirmation approach claim that puberty suppressors constitute "Fully reversible therapy that suspends pubertal development."[26] And second, as Abel explains, "Pubertal suppression allows, many argue, for optimal results of the potential cross-gender transition, as secondary sex characteristics of one's natal

---

24. Kuper, "Puberty Blocking Medications," 2.

25. Hruz et al., "Growing Pains," 10–11.

26. Giovanardi, "Buying Time or Arresting Development?," 154.

sex are difficult to undo."[27] Early preparation for gender transition is the ultimate goal of puberty suppression under the gender affirmation model, as Cretella observes: "The suffering of transgender adults was invoked to argue for the urgent rescue of children from the same fate by early identification, affirmation, and pubertal suppression."[28] In summary, advocates of the gender affirming approach maintain that puberty-suppressing hormones make gender transition easier and more convincing for children whose gender dysphoria persists through adulthood. From the moment puberty suppression begins, the goal is gender transition for all children who undergo this treatment plan.

Now, concerning the oft-maligned terms of "persistence" and "desistance," Zucker explains, "The terms persistence and desistance became part of the linguistic landscape with regard to children with a diagnosis of . . . gender dysphoria."[29] While Giovanardi acknowledges that research on gender-dysphoric children is sparse, he reports:

> It is now acknowledged, for instance, that children's GD/ GV persists after puberty in only 10–30 per cent of all cases; when it does not, the children are referred to as "desisters." At present, there is no way to predict which individuals will or will not suffer from GD into adolescence or adulthood. However, "persisters," whose GD continues into adolescence, are more likely to experience GD in adulthood.[30]

Even the most ardent proponents of gender affirmation must admit that, based on current desistance rates, if the child is simply left untreated, the distress associated with gender dysphoria will cease in the majority of children. Furthermore, gender affirmation advocates also admit that it is impossible to identify which gender-dysphoric children will persist and which ones will desist. Therefore, since the majority of gender-dysphoric and TGNC children

27. Abel, "Hormone Treatment of Children," S24.
28. Cretella, "Gender Dysphoria in Children," 52.
29. Zucker, "Myth of Persistence," 232.
30. Giovanardi, "Buying Time or Arresting Development?," 153.

will desist, it is vital for individuals such as parents, medical practitioners, and ministry professionals to serve as gatekeepers for unnecessary medical intervention.

Beauchamp and Childress ascribe the ethically necessary role of gatekeeper to those with the authority to distinguish, "Persons whose decisions should be . . . accepted from persons whose decisions . . . should not be . . . accepted."[31] Implicit in this definition is the understanding that some medical requests should not be affirmed because they are harmful, unjust, unnecessary, or unethical. However, with the rise to prominence of the gender affirmation approach, gatekeeping garners mostly negative connotations in contemporary culture. Puckett et al. associate medical gatekeeping with bias and transphobia due to the fact that it leaves TGNC individuals feeling, "Disempowered and with few resources to overcome such challenges."[32] Singal expounds on the moral conflict facing medical professionals who attempt to practice ethical gatekeeping in an affirmation-dominated climate, reporting:

> Clinicians are still wrestling with how to define affirming care, and how to balance affirmation and caution when treating adolescents. "I don't want to be a gatekeeper," Dianne Berg, a co-director of the National Center for Gender Spectrum Health, at the University of Minnesota, told me. "But I also worry that in opening the gates, we're going to have more adolescents that don't engage in the reflective work needed in order to make sound decisions, and there might end up being more people when they are older that are like, Oh, hmm—now I am not sure about this."[33]

As the significance of gatekeeping wanes, the pressure for the universal acceptance of gender-affirming care is mounting. For example, parents of gender-dysphoric or TGNC children who believe that their child's gender expression and gender identity are truly incongruent with their natal gender can affirm their child's

---

31. Beauchamp and Childress, *Principles of Biomedical Ethics*, 114.

32. Puckett et al., "Barriers to Gender-affirming Care," 56.

33. Singal, "Your Child Says She's Trans," 97.

desired gender by seeking gender confirmation surgery.[34] This process begins with a visit to one of the many new gender clinics now operating in the USA, where GnRH agonists can be legally prescribed for off-label use in order to interrupt puberty.[35] Gender affirmation also includes such social behaviors as issuing a rebirth announcement in anticipation of gender transition.[36] Presently, puberty suppression as recommended by gender affirmation practitioners is becoming a common practice for treating gender-dysphoric and TGNC children.[37] Furthermore, as a result of increased pressure and popularity in both politics and culture, the demands for unrestricted access to puberty-suppressing hormones will likely increase in the near future.[38] So the question at hand for parents, medical providers, and ministry professionals is not whether puberty can be suppressed, but rather, should this course of action be pursued? Does the administration of puberty-suppressing hormones constitute ethical treatment of gender-dysphoric and TGNC children? Is gender affirmation an acceptable treatment plan for gender-dysphoric children? The best way to begin to answer these questions is to analyze what happens during puberty.

34. Sifferlin, "Gender Confirmation Surgery." Formerly known as "sex change" or "sexual reassignment surgery" (SRS), the procedure has been renamed in order to be more positive and affirming.

35. Cretella, "Gender Dysphoria in Children," 52. Cretella notes that the first gender clinic for children opened in Boston in 2007, and by 2016, forty other clinics had opened across the country.

36. Sieczkowski, "Mom's Birth Announcement."

37. Hruz et al., "Growing Pains," 5.

38. Cretella, "Gender Dysphoria in Children," 52. Cretella observes, "In 2014 there were 24 gender clinics clustered chiefly along the East coast and in California; one year later there were 40 across the nation. Dr Ximena Lopes . . . stated, '[Use of this protocol is] growing really fast. And the main reason is [that] parents are demanding it'" (52).

3

What Happens in Puberty?

BY NOW YOU MAY be wondering, "What exactly happens during puberty that is so disturbing to gender-dysphoric and TGNC children?" The main cause of distress is the development of gender-specific primary and secondary sexual characteristics that are stimulated by the human body's production of GnRH. These characteristics make natal males more masculine and natal females more feminine. GnRH agonists, also known as puberty suppressors, interfere with the body's production of GnRH and, as a result, impede the development of primary and secondary sexual characteristics. In order to appreciate how GnRH agonists function, it is imperative to consider the systemic changes that occur to the human body during puberty.

Puberty-suppressing hormones are designed to interrupt the biochemical function of the endocrine system of children during the early stages of adolescence. The endocrine system contains the glands that produce hormones. By impeding the endocrine system and intentionally interfering with the development of children, these chemicals have far-reaching effects on the human body. Ward and Hisley explain:

> The endocrine system is composed of multiple organs throughout the body. These organs secrete hormones

that regulate various bodily functions . . . The endocrine system controls growth and development as well as energy use and energy stores; it also controls levels of sugar, salt, and fluids in the bloodstream. [1]

The endocrine system is comprised primarily of the hypothalamus, pituitary gland, thyroid gland, adrenal glands, pancreas, pineal gland, and parathyroid glands; and it also includes hormones secreted from the heart, thymus, digestive tract, kidneys, and gonads.[2] Therefore, the endocrine system is not a closed or isolated system, but rather a complex system that interacts with all other systems of the human body. This means that the use of GnRH agonists will not just inhibit a natal female's breast development or a natal male's Adam's apple, but will have sweeping consequences to their brain and body.

The three main components of the endocrine system that are directly affected by puberty-suppressing hormones are the hypothalamus, the pituitary gland, and the gonads. Both the hypothalamus and the pituitary gland are located deep within the brain. Technically, the hypothalamus, which naturally produces GnRH during puberty,[3] is located between the thalamus and the pituitary gland in the central region of the brain known as the diencephalon.[4] Martini et al. describe the diencephalon as, "The structural and functional link between the cerebral hemispheres and the rest of the CNS [central nervous system] . . . The hypothalamus . . . or floor of the diencephalon, contains centers involved with emotions, autonomic function, and hormone production."[5] Autonomic function controlled by the hypothalamus includes regulating body temperature, thirst, body weight, appetite, sex drive, blood pressure, and heart rate.[6] Puberty suppression focuses on masking the hormone production function of the hypothalamus that acts on

1. Ward et al., *Maternal-Child Nursing Care*, 1060.

2. Martini et al., *Visual Anatomy and Physiology*, 589.

3. Martini et al., *Visual Anatomy and Physiology*, 594.

4. Johnson, "What is the Function?"

5. Martini et al., *Visual Anatomy and Physiology*, 464.

6. Johnson, "What is the Function?"

the pituitary gland. Johnson explains, "The hypothalamus is close-ly related to the pituitary gland . . . Together the hypothalamus and pituitary gland work to control the entire endocrine system."[7]

The pituitary gland rests below the hypothalamus in the sphenoid bone of the skull. The anterior lobe of the pituitary gland responds to GnRH by producing the dual gonadotropins Follicle-stimulating hormone (FSH) and Luteinizing hormone (LH), respectively. Martini et al. describe the function of the pituitary gland as follows:

> Nine important peptide hormones are released by the pituitary gland—seven by the anterior lobe and two by the posterior lobe . . . The hormones of the anterior lobe are also called tropic hormones, because they 'turn on' endocrine glands or support the functions of other or-gans . . . The hormones called gonadotropins regulate the activities of the gonads.[8]

FSH and LH are the tropic hormones that control the de-velopment of the gonads. Martini et al. explain that, "The gonads produce gametes and hormones."[9] In natal males, both gametes and hormones are produced in the testes. This includes the pro-duction of sperm and androgens (testosterone).[10] In natal females, both gametes and hormones are produced in the ovaries. This includes the maturation of eggs and production of estrogens.[11] Puberty-suppressing hormones are designed to counteract the function of both the hypothalamus and the pituitary gland in the brain in order to prevent the production or maturation of gametes and hormones in the gonads. This interruption of normal func-tion ultimately inhibits the development of primary and second-ary sexual characteristics during adolescence. Therefore, parents and children alike must understand that GnRH agonists primarily

7. Martini et al., *Visual Anatomy and Physiology*, 464.

8. Martini et al., *Visual Anatomy and Physiology*, 594.

9. Martini et al., *Visual Anatomy and Physiology*, 989.

10. Martini et al., *Visual Anatomy and Physiology*, 989.

11. Martini et al., *Visual Anatomy and Physiology*, 1003.

target and affect the brain of the developing child, which in turn affects the gonads, which in turn affects the rest of the body.

Puberty describes the period of transition from childhood to adulthood also known as adolescence.[12] Ward and Hisley explain that, "Adolescence technically begins with the onset of puberty when the pituitary gland relays messages to sex glands to manufacture hormones necessary for reproduction."[13] Kuper outlines the systemic effects of puberty on the human body, stating, "Puberty involves changes in body structures, body functions, and physical appearance."[14] These changes, summarized by Hruz et al., include a growth spurt, the development of primary and secondary sex characteristics, and, "Changes in body composition."[15] Progression through puberty is measured visibly by a system of Tanner staging I–V. Kuper explains:

> Individuals at Tanner stage I are pre-pubertal, meaning they have not yet experienced any pubertal changes. Tanner stage II reflects the start of puberty, while stage III and IV reflect continued pubertal changes. By Tanner stage V, sex characteristics have reached adult development. Tanner stages are typically assessed via examination of breast size, testicular volume and penis size, and pubic hair.[16]

In both natal males and females, the development of primary and secondary sex characteristics beginning late in Tanner stage II ultimately result in a greater anatomical distinction between the genders. Furthermore, this is the point where the ability to reproduce is achieved.[17] While puberty-suppressing hormones do counteract some anatomical distinctions, including the ability to reproduce, they do not suspend every aspect of puberty. At best, GnRH agonists can achieve partial suppression of puberty.

12. Martini et al., *Visual Anatomy and Physiology*, 1047.

13. Ward et al., *Maternal-Child Nursing Care*, 780–81.

14. Kuper, "Puberty Blocking Medications," 2.

15. Hruz et al., "Growing Pains," 7.

16. Kuper, "Puberty Blocking Medications," 2.

17. Kuper, "Puberty Blocking Medications," 7.

From a biochemical perspective, Hruz et al. explain that progression through puberty is determined by the successive release of three different hormones in the human body.[18] These hormones include androgens, GnRH, and human growth hormone (GH) respectively.[19] Hruz et al. further reveal that scientists mark the chemical onset of puberty with the "Beginning of adrenal maturation."[20] This process, which commences between ages six and nine in natal females, and seven and ten in natal males, occurs when the adrenal glands produce androgens that result in the shared physical outcomes of "Oily skin, acne, body odor, and the growth of axillary and pubic hair."[21] Adrenal maturation typically marks the beginning of Tanner stage II and is followed by "Gonadal maturation."[22] This process occurs between the ages of eight and thirteen in natal females, and nine and fourteen in natal males, when the release of GnRH from the hypothalamus results in "The development of the basic reproductive capacity and external sex characteristics that distinguish the sexes."[23] Gonadal maturation begins late in Tanner stage II and continues through Tanner stage IV. The third and final biochemical factor of puberty involves the "Increased production of human growth hormone."[24] This process, which typically occurs after adrenal and gonadal maturation are underway and interacts with the hormones released in both stages, results in major physiological changes that include a growth spurt, changes in bone density and fat distribution, hair growth, and gonad maturation.[25] All three biochemical processes of puberty are interrelated. GnRH agonists interrupt one of these three processes. The long-term effects of suspending gonadal maturation in children, while allowing adrenal maturation to continue unimpeded

18. Hruz et al., "Growing Pains," 8–9.

19. Hruz et al., "Growing Pains," 8–9.

20. Hruz et al., "Growing Pains," 8–9.

21. Hruz et al., "Growing Pains," 8–9.

22. Hruz et al., "Growing Pains," 8–9.

23. Hruz et al., "Growing Pains," 8–9.

24. Hruz et al., "Growing Pains," 8–9.

25. Hruz et al., "Growing Pains," 8–9.

and the growth phase to continue partially impeded, has dangerous implications.

In conclusion, puberty consists of much more than the development of primary and secondary sexual characteristics. The human brain, musculoskeletal system, and internal organs all undergo significant changes and growth during adolescence. Synthetically interrupting part of this process in gender-dysphoric and TGNC children in order to produce purely cosmetic alterations for an unknown percentage of individuals who may persist is not only ethically suspect, but is damaging to the long-term health and well-being of the individual. And yet, this is the course of treatment mandated by advocates of gender affirmation. The systemic effects of puberty-suppressing hormones will be examined in greater detail in the following chapter.

4

How is Puberty Suppressed?

IF YOUR CHILD IS petitioning for puberty-suppressing hormones, then as a parent, you have a responsibility to learn what puberty-suppressing hormones will do to the developing body of your child. In short, puberty-suppressing hormones interfere with the production of GnRH in the brain. Due to the fact that the natural release of GnRH by the hypothalamus during gonadal maturation directly influences the development of the primary and secondary sexual characteristics, which, in turn, causes distress to gender-dysphoric and TGNC children, puberty-suppressing hormones known as GnRH agonists are intended to counter the natural effects of GnRH on the pituitary gland. GnRH agonists are currently administered to children as early as Tanner stage II in order to prevent the development of primary and secondary sexual characteristics.[1] Hruz et al. describe the chemical process that occurs during gonadal maturation as follows:

> Specialized neurons in the hypothalamus secrete . . .
> GnRH . . . The hypothalamus releases bursts of GnRH,
> and when the pituitary gland is exposed to these bursts,
> it responds by secreting two other hormones. These

1. Cretella, "Gender Dysphoria in Children," 52. This indicates that children as young as eight years old have begun the transition process under gender-affirming care with the consent of parents and medical professionals.

are luteinizing hormone (LH) and follicle-stimulating hormone (FSH), which stimulate the growth of the gonads . . . In addition to regulating the maturation of the gonads and the production of sex hormones, these two hormones also play an important role in regulating aspects of human fertility.[2]

Since it is the burst, or fluctuating levels of GnRH, that ultimately triggers the pituitary gland to release LH and FSH, high doses of synthetic GnRH are administered on a regular basis to patients wishing to suppress puberty. By maintaining a constant blood level of GnRH, doctors are able to prevent the maturation of the gonads, which in turn impedes the development of primary and secondary sex characteristics. Hruz et al. explain: "The additional GnRH 'desensitizes' the pituitary, leading to a decrease in the secretions of . . . LH and FSH, which in turn leads to a decreased maturation of and secretion of sex hormones by gonads."[3]

At this point, it is necessary to make four observations regarding the administration of GnRH agonists. First, gender-dysphoric or TGNC children who wish to prevent the development of primary and secondary sexual characteristics must be given large doses of synthetic hormones over long periods of time during a crucial stage of physical and emotional development. This fact is uncontested by gender affirmation advocates such as WPATH. The administration of puberty-suppressing hormones can begin as early as ages eight to ten and are ultimately supplemented with the respective cross-sex hormone estrogen or testosterone. GnRH agonists act directly on the pituitary gland in the brain, essentially tricking the body by masking the natural bursts of GnRH produced by the hypothalamus with a continuous, elevated level of GnRH. The long-term effects of these synthetic hormones on the hypothalamus, pituitary gland, or rest of the human body remain unknown. Cretella reports on the claims of evidence-based medicine as follows:

> There is not a single large, randomized, controlled study that documents the alleged benefits and potential harms

---

2. Hruz et al., "Growing Pains," 8–9.

3. Hruz et al., "Growing Pains," 8–9.

to gender-dysphoric children from pubertal suppression and decades of cross-sex hormone use. Nor is there a single long-term, large, randomized, controlled study that compares the outcomes of various psychotherapeutic interventions for childhood GD with those of pubertal suppression followed by decades of toxic synthetic steroids . . . Pubertal suppression at Tanner Stage 2 followed by the use of cross-sex hormones will leave these children sterile.[4]

Second, while GnRH agonists will prevent the development of primary and secondary sexual characteristics, contrary to Kuper, they do not halt puberty. Nor do they stop time.[5] Nor do they alter the child's natal or biological gender. With regard to puberty, while GnRH agonists will prevent gonadal maturation and impede the release the HGH, they will not inhibit adrenal maturation. Therefore, the terms, "Partially suppressed puberty" or "Puberty interfering hormones" better describe the effects of GnRH agonists on human development, since some aspects of the maturation process are artificially stunted while the rest continue to develop. This, too, is an uncontested fact. However, this is also problematic for the long-term health of the child, since gonadal maturation is not an isolated process in human development. Other areas of development will be affected by the long-term use of synthetic puberty suppressors.

Third, with regard to gender transition from male to female (MtF) or female to male (FtM), Cretella explains the significance of a biblical and scientific gender binary:

Sex chromosome pairs 'XY' and 'XX' are genetic markers of sex, male, and female, respectively. They are not genetic markers of a disordered body or birth defect. Human sexuality is binary by design, with the purpose of being the reproduction of our species . . . Barring one of the rare disorders of sex development, no infant is 'assigned'

4. Cretella, "Gender Dysphoria in Children and Suppression of Debate," 52.

5. Hruz et al., "Growing Pains," 12.

a sex a birth; rather birth sex declares itself anatomically in utero and is acknowledged at birth.[6]

Therefore, no amount of puberty suppression, cross-sex hormone treatment, sexual reassignment/corrective surgeries, or gender affirmation can actually change the gender of a human being. Like the previous two observations, this fact is irrefutable. For, as Cretella states, "From a purely scientific standpoint, human beings possess a biologically predetermined sex and innate sex differences . . . Sex change is objectively impossible."[7] At best, transition procedures beginning with GnRH agonists, even when supplemented with all other aspects of gender affirmation, can only provide an elaborate, expensive, painful, irreversible, and incomplete disguise that will require a lifetime of maintenance to sustain.

Finally, Cretella explains that the use of GnRH agonists to suppress puberty in gender-dysphoric and TGNC children does have adverse side effects, including the fact that these hormones, "Arrest bone growth, decrease bone accretion, prevent the sex-steroid dependent organization and maturation of the adolescent brain, and inhibit fertility by preventing the development of gonadal tissue and mature gametes for the duration of treatment."[8] Nonetheless, whether or not it is dangerous to bathe a developing child's brain with high doses of synthetic hormones for over a decade is often challenged by gender affirmation advocates, and more information will likely become available as the first generation to be administered GnRH agonists continues to age. However, the harmful effects of GnRH agonists are compounded with the administration of cross-sex hormones which, while producing the desired secondary sexual characteristics in gender-dysphoric and TGNC children, also results in infertility and long-term health issues after puberty. The adverse effects of cross-sex hormones on the human body are not debated, and under gender affirmation puberty suppression leads directly to cross-sex hormone therapy.

6. Cretella, "Gender Dysphoria in Children and Suppression of Debate," 51.

7. Cretella, "Gender Dysphoria in Children," 289.

8. Cretella, "Gender Dysphoria in Children and Suppression of Debate," 53.

5

What Happens to Gender-dysphoric Children after Puberty?

IF A GENDER-DYSPHORIC OR TGNC child is administered puberty-suppressing hormones during adolescence in order to prevent the development of primary and secondary sexual characteristics, then the next reasonable question to ask is, "What happens after puberty? Does the gender dysphoric individual remain in a state of suspended development indefinitely?" The answer is, no. The truth of the matter is that the gender affirmation process guides the child toward gender transition, beginning with puberty suppression that leads to harmful cross-sex hormone therapy and ultimately to sexual reassignment surgeries. For children pursuing gender transition, cross-sex hormone therapy is typically initiated at Tanner stage V, normally around age sixteen. Cross-sex hormone therapy includes the administration of testosterone for females and estrogens for males. However, Cretella reports that some gender affirmation specialists are now, "Putting children as young as 11 years old directly onto cross-sex hormones."[1] Such radical gender-affirming treatment on a young child would, for example, cause an eleven-year-old natal male to develop breasts and be rendered

---

1. Cretella, "Gender Dysphoria in Children," 296.

infertile without taking into consideration either the possibility of desistance or the potentially devastating effects to the long-term physical health of the child.

While experts debate whether or not the effects of puberty-suppressing hormones are reversible, the general consensus of both advocates and critics of the gender affirmation method is that effects of cross-sex hormones are irreversible. Along with the intended results of infertility and the partial development of some secondary sexual characteristics of the opposite natal gender, Cretella explains that the unintended health risks associated with cross-sex hormones also include,

> Thrombosis, cardiovascular disease, weight gain, hyper-trigyceridemia, elevated blood pressure, decreased glucose tolerance, gallbladder disease, prolactinoma, breast cancer . . . low HDL and elevated tryglycerides, increased homocysteine levels, hepatotoxicity, polycynthemia, increased risk of sleep apnea, and insulin resistance.[2]

Even WPATH's *Standards of Care*, which purports to provide guidelines for gender affirmation therapy, recognizes the permanent nature of cross-sex hormone treatment. While technically labeling cross-sex estrogen and testosterone therapy as partially reversible treatments,[3] the authors of WPATH later admit that, "Feminizing/masculinizing hormone therapy may lead to irreversible physical changes."[4]

Chemical transition alone, even when implemented early with puberty suppression, supplemented with cross-sex hormone therapy, enhanced with social factors such as hair and clothes styles, and aided by gender affirmation, is not the final step in the transition process. Sexual reassignment surgery (SRS), now argued medically necessary for corrective measures by gender affirmation advocates,[5] is the next phase in the transition process that begins

---

2. Cretella, "Gender Dysphoria in Children and Suppression of Debate," 53.

3. Coleman et al., "Standards of Care," 19.

4. Coleman et al., "Standards of Care," 36.

5. Coleman et al., "Standards of Care," 54.

with puberty-suppressing hormones. SRS includes a vast array of painful, complicated, and expensive top and bottom surgeries that permanently alter the body and require a lifetime of maintenance in order to maintain the illusion of gender transition.

6

Why Were Puberty Suppressors Invented in the First Place?

BY NOW YOU MAY have more questions than answers. These next few chapters are intended to anticipate some of those questions while continuing to evaluate whether or not the use of GnRH agonists constitutes ethical treatment of gender-dysphoric and TGNC children. First, you may wonder, "If puberty-suppressing hormones are so dangerous, then why were they created in the first place?" Puberty-suppressing hormones were originally developed to treat precocious puberty, not gender dysphoria.[1] As Cretella observes, the major difference between these two conditions lies in the fact that precocious puberty is a documented physical condition, while gender dysphoria is a purely psychological condition.[2] If precocious puberty is not suppressed, children will face serious health problems from premature gonadal maturation. Analyzing the difference between precocious puberty and gender dysphoria helps explain why puberty-suppressing hormones are appropriate for the former and dangerous for the latter.

1. Hruz et al., "Growing Pains," 10.
2. Cretella, "Gender Dysphoria in Children and Suppression of Debate," 50.

For children with precocious puberty, gonadal maturation begins prematurely. Therefore, children diagnosed with precocious puberty are typically placed on GnRH agonists until they reach the normal age for puberty onset based on their natal gender. For example, a four-year-old natal female who begins to experience gonadal maturation would be placed on GnRH agonists until she reaches the age of approximately eight or nine. At such time, after adrenal maturation has commenced in her body, GnRH agonists would be discontinued, and normal puberty would resume. The benefits of temporarily administering GnRH agonists to children with precocious puberty far outweigh the side effects. Furthermore, any evidence cited by gender affirmation proponents to support the safe and reversible claims of GnRH agonists pertains only to the treatment of children with precocious puberty, not to the treatment of gender dysphoria in otherwise healthy children. Singal admits, "Data about the potential risks of putting young people on puberty blockers are scarce."[3] GnRH agonists have neither been tested nor approved for treatment of gender dysphoria in children, and therefore constitute an off-label, experimental use.

In summary, proponents of gender affirmation advocate for the prescription of GnRH agonists in order to prevent the development of primary and secondary sexual characteristics in gender-dysphoric and TGNC children. These advocates appeal to the successful hormone treatment of children with precocious puberty in order to justify the use of GnRH agonists for gender-dysphoric and TGNC children. However, there are several major differences between precocious puberty and gender dysphoria that are ignored in this assumption. First, the ultimate treatment goal for children with precocious puberty is to normalize human development as much as possible. In contrast, the goal of prescribing GnRH agonists to TGNC children under the gender affirmation model is to disrupt human development as much as possible. This disruption prepares the child's body for cross-sex hormone therapy and gender transition surgeries. Second, in precocious puberty, GnRH agonists are prescribed to correct a physical disorder. In

---

3. Singal, "Your Child Says She's Trans," 94.

gender-dysphoric and TGNC children, GnRH agonists are administered in order to arrest normal physical development, thereby creating a physical disorder. Finally, GnRH agonists are discontinued for children with precocious puberty when they reach the normal age for gonadal maturation. For gender-dysphoric children, GnRH agonists are not administered until they reach the age of normal gonadal maturation, and they continue indefinitely or until the gonads are surgically removed. If the gender-dysphoric or TGNC child elects to keep their gonads after Tanner stage V, the child will be sterile, but they will still need to remain on a combination of GnRH agonists and cross-sex hormones for the remainder of their lives. The long-term effects of this treatment method on an otherwise physically healthy natal male or female is unknown due to a lack of scientific testing.

7

What Causes Gender Dysphoria in Children?

BY NOW YOU ARE likely wondering, "Why? Why is my child, my patient, or my student struggling with their gender identity?" Etiology, the search for a cause, represents one of several areas where a general consensus concerning gender-dysphoric and TGNC children exists. Yarhouse concisely summarizes the prevailing view as follows: "We do not know what causes gender dysphoria."[1] In short, all sides presently agree that all possible causes of gender nonconformity and its associated distress are not currently known. However, as the increased reliance on GnRH agonists indicates, the lack of understanding as to why gender dysphoria occurs in children does not preclude radical treatment options. Hruz et al. explain that most gender affirming proponents approach gender-dysphoric and TGNC children with the following mindset: "Treating gender dysphoria does not require us first to understand its causes."[2] This is a dangerous approach. Hruz et al. counter this logic by explaining the importance of recognizing

1. Yarhouse, *Understanding Gender Dysphoria*, 61.
2. Hruz et al., "Growing Pains," 15.

how underlying conditions either contribute to or complicate a current state of distress.[3]

In support of Hruz et al., recent research has revealed that a variety of underlying conditions often do exist for gender dysphoria. For example, a 2010 study by de Vries et al. confirmed that Autism Spectrum Disorder (ASD) "occurs more frequently in gender dysphoric individuals than expected by chance,"[4] particularly in natal males.[5] Furthermore, Firth reports that "clinical experience with such clients is freighted with personal histories of abuse and neglect, often combined with common, sometimes extreme, mental health problems."[6] Firth proceeds to examine a case of a gender-dysphoric natal female who was sexually abused multiple times by a teenage male babysitter at age nine as a typical example of a TGNC client.[7] This is not to imply that every gender-dysphoric or TGNC child is a sexual assault survivor or falls on the autism spectrum, but it does indicate that GnRH agonists may mask or even aggravate the true underlying problem, which could range from autism to mental illness to a traumatic experience. The etiological debate primarily concerns whether gender identity issues are physically innate (nature) or environmentally learned (nurture) behaviors.

In the age-old debate of nature vs. nurture, brain-sex theories take the side of nature by seeking to identify a physical cause for gender dysphoria that is associated with the brain.[8] For example, the popular acceptance of these theories by advocates of the gender affirmation approach is evident in the contemporary catch-phrasing of a TGNC natal male as possessing a, "female brain in a male body," and vice versa.[9] Yarhouse identifies the two leading

---

3. Hruz et al., "Growing Pains," 15.

4. de Vries et al., "Autism Spectrum Disorders," 933. The de Vries et al. study is recognized and recorded in WPATH's *Standards of Care*, 12–13.

5. de Vries et al., "Autism Spectrum Disorders," 934.

6. Firth, "Childhood Abuse and Depressive Vulnerability," 297.

7. Firth, "Childhood Abuse and Depressive Vulnerability," 301.

8. Yarhouse, *Understanding Gender Dysphoria*, 73.

9. Cretella, "Gender Dysphoria in Children and Suppression of Debate," 51.

brain-sex candidates as the "prenatal hormone hypothesis . . . (and the)... neuroanatomic brain differences hypothesis."[10]

Advocates for the prenatal hormone hypothesis speculate that a female embryo's exposure to increased levels of testosterone or a male embryo's exposure to increased levels of estrogen while in the uterus predisposes a child to gender dysphoria. To this line of thinking, Yarhouse gently observes, "There is research that does not appear to support the theory."[11] With the exception of the intersex condition known as Androgen Insensitivity Syndrome (AIS), natal males secrete and absorb testosterone in utero, while natal females lack the ability to produce testosterone. Therefore, the prenatal hormone premise is both untenable and untestable.

While prenatal hormone hypothesis appeals to chemical factors in order to explain gender dysphoria in children, the neuroanatomic brain difference hypothesis argues for a variation in brain structure. The structure of the hypothalamus is currently the focal point of study.[12] But, like the prenatal hormone hypothesis, the theory of an innate brain structure variation in gender-dysphoric children is not congruent with the evidence, the strongest of which is the result of twin studies.

If biological factors such as embryonic exposure to hormones in the uterus or brain structure variation were primarily responsible for gender dysphoria, then TGNC monozygotic twins should offer the strongest evidence to support this hypothesis, since both would have been exposed to the same hormones in utero and possess the same genetic make-up for brain structure. Therefore, gender-dysphoric and TGNC rates should be identical 100 percent of the time in monozygotic twins. However, as Cretella reports:

> Regarding etiology of transgenderism, twin studies of adult transsexuals prove definitively that prenatal genetic and hormone influence is minimal . . . Only 21 monozygotic twin pairs out of a total of 74 monozygotic pairs . . . were concordant for transsexualism . . . This means that

10. Yarhouse, *Understanding Gender Dysphoria*, 67–68.

11. Yarhouse, *Understanding Gender Dysphoria*, 68.

12. Yarhouse, *Understanding Gender Dysphoria*, 68.

at least 72 percent of what accounts for transsexualism in one twin and not in the other occurs after birth and is not biological. Such a high discordance rate among identical twins proves that no one is born pre-determined to have gender dysphoria.[13]

Notably, the discordance rates of monozygotic twins are consistent with the general desistance rate of TGNC children. However, a glaring lack of scientific evidence has not prevented radical gender affirming advocates from operating under the assumption that brain-sex theory will ultimately be proven true. For example, Meier and Harris report, "Although no consensus exists on the etiology of gender diversity, neurobiological evidence for sex-specific brain differences in transgender people is being explored."[14] Meier and Harris then conclude, "One's gender identity is very resistant, if not immutable, to any type of environmental intervention."[15] Ironically, Meier and Harris's statement is not only contested by critics of the gender affirmation approach, but it is directly contradicted by some of the most ardent proponents of gender affirmation who insist that gender identity is in fact mutable. For example, leading gender affirmation advocates Temple Newhook et al. contend, "Gender identity can indeed shift and evolve over time."[16] This statement supports evangelical scholar Armand Nicholi Jr., who explains: "Social and psychological factors such as our early life experiences determine our gender identity."[17] Therefore, in order to make the assertion that gender identity is solely biologically-based and immutable, gender affirmation proponents such as Meier and Harris must disregard desistance rates, operate under the presupposition that brain-sex theory is correct, and ignore the scientific phenomenon of neuroplasticity.

Concerning neuroplasticity, Cretella explains: "Neuroplasticity is the well-established phenomenon in which long-term

13. Cretella, "Gender Dysphoria in Children," 290.

14. Meier and Harris, "Fact Sheet," para. 4.

15. Meier and Harris, "Fact Sheet," para. 4.

16. Temple Newhook et al., "Critical Commentary," 214.

17. Nicholi, "Human Sexuality," 341–42.

behavior alters brain microstructures."[18] Wesson confirms that physical changes in the brain are created by environmental factors, stating, "Our brains undergo daily renovations to adapt to our ever-changing world."[19] These changes, which can be brought on by injury, drug use, traumatic experiences, or repeated behavior over time, include the creation or elimination of neural pathways that actually alter the physical structure of the brain along with the thinking process of the individual. This phenomenon allows Cretella to assert, "If and when valid transgender brain differences are identified, these will likely be the result of transgender behavior rather than its cause."[20] Hruz et al. support Cretella's hypothesis and, contra Meier and Harris who insist that gender identity is fixed, confirm, "Gender identity for children is elastic (that is, it can change over time) and plastic (that is, it can be shaped by forces like parental approval and social conditions)."[21] Therefore, the evidence points to the fact that environmental factors can and do significantly influence one's gender identity. In short, if you take a prepubescent cisgender natal male, force him to dress like a female, change his name to a female name, treat him like a female, and administer hormones that suppress his masculine features, Meier and Harris insist that he will never question whether or not he is a male, while Cretella and Hruz maintain that he can become confused about his gender or even convinced that he is a female over time. Both science and common sense seem to support Cretella and Hruz.

Contrary to brain-sex theory, advocates of the therapeutic model of treatment generally seek an explanation for gender dysphoria derived primarily from environmental factors. Cretella explains the variation in transgender twin studies as follows:

> Non-shared post-natal events . . . predominate in the development and persistence of gender dysphoria in one twin verses the other. This is not surprising since it is

18. Cretella, "Gender Dysphoria in Children," 289.

19. Wesson, "Primer on Neuroplasticity," para. 3.

20. Cretella, "Gender Dysphoria in Children," 289–90.

21. Hruz et al., "Growing Pains," 6.

well accepted that a child's emotional and psychological development is impacted by positive and negative experiences from infancy forward. Family and peer relationships, one's school and neighborhood, the experience of any form of abuse, media exposure, chronic illness, war and natural disasters are all examples of environmental factors that impact an individual's emotional, social, and psychological development.[22]

Firth confirms Cretella's assertions, reporting:

> Psychological and family-based studies provide moderate evidence of transwomen having more cold, controlling or rejecting fathers . . . more brothers than sisters and later birth order . . . and of transmen having cold or rejecting parents and over-controlling mothers . . . Similarly, supporters of family-based studies observe that mentally ill parents are more likely to seek help for their GV offspring[23]

While Yarhouse is quick to point out that these environmental factors are correlative,[24] the shared experiences of gender-dysphoric and TGNC children do provide etiological insights. Cretella lists several determinative factors, including social media binging, sexual abuse, and the dysfunctional family dynamics of physical abuse, emotional abuse, and neglect as aggravating gender dysphoria. Singal confirms, "Trauma, particularly sexual trauma, can contribute to or exacerbate dysphoria in some patients, but again, no one yet knows exactly why."[25] These shared elements are all frequently documented in the lives of gender-dysphoric and TGNC children.[26] To these contributing environmental influences, Yarhouse adds that physical similarities with the opposite gender, a parental preference for the opposite gender child, and peer influences are also factors that can affect developing gender

22. Cretella, "Gender Dysphoria in Children," 291.
23. Firth, "Childhood Abuse and Depressive Vulnerability," 100.
24. Yarhouse, *Understanding Gender Dysphoria*, 77.
25. Singal, "Your Child Says She's Trans," 94.
26. Cretella, "Gender Dysphoria in Children," 292–93.

identity.[27] Drescher and Pula further note the impact that environmental factors have on the development of gender dysphoria, suggesting, "GD/GV may be mimicked by gender confusion that occurs . . . as a result of sexual trauma or delusions in the context of psychotic disorders."[28] Therefore, while the general consensus agrees that there does not exist any one etiological explanation for every presentation of gender dysphoria in children, any legitimate evidence-based approach must take environmental factors into consideration. And, if the gender dysphoria is in fact a result of environmental factors such as physical or sexual abuse, media influence, or dysfunctional family dynamics, then it is reasonable to conclude that the distress the child is experiencing will not be alleviated by a long-term synthetic hormone regiment intended to suppress puberty.

Another area of general consensus regarding gender dysphoria in children concerns the phenomenon of desistance. Drescher and Pula explain, "The gender dysphoria of the majority of children with GD/GV does not persist into adolescence, and when it does not, the children are referred to as 'desisters.'"[29] Cretella reports, "80 percent to 95 percent of pre-pubertal children with GD will experience resolution by late adolescence if not exposed to social affirmation and medical intervention."[30] Children who continue to present symptoms consistent with gender dysphoria are labeled persisters. There is some statistical discrepancy among experts concerning persistence rates. For example, Hruz et al. cite the persistence rates as recorded in DSM as 2.2 to 30 percent in natal males and 12 to 50 percent in natal females;[31] Giovanardi reports that 10 to 30 percent of gender-dysphoric children in general will persist;[32] Ristori and Steensma document the overall persis-

27. Yarhouse, *Understanding Gender Dysphoria*, 77.
28. Dresher and Pula, "Ethical Issues Raised," S18.
29. Dresher and Pula, "Ethical Issues Raised," S18.
30. Cretella, "Gender Dysphoria in Children," 298.
31. Hruz et al., "Growing Pains," 19.
32. Giovanardi, "Buying Time or Arresting Development?," 153.

tence rates between 2 to 39 percent;[33] and WPATH's *Standards of Care* recognizes that persistence rates range from 6 to 23 percent.[34] Common ground can be found in the fact that nearly all experts, including the most ardent advocates of gender affirmation such as WPATH, recognize that in the overwhelming majority of cases, if not affirmed, the distress associated with gender dysphoria does eventually desist in children.

Desistance rates factor prominently in treatment methods. Proponents of the therapeutic model argue that individual and family therapy facilitates desistance. Advocates of a watchful waiting approach maintain that the symptoms will eventually subside if not affirmed. Meanwhile, Temple Newhook et al. insist that failure to provide gender affirmation for persisters results in, "Harm when attempting to delay or defer transition."[35] However, Drescher and Pula reveal that the problem with the underlying assumption of the gender affirmation approach lies in the fact that, "There is at present no way to predict in which children GD/GV will or will not persist into adulthood."[36] Later, the same authors insist, "There are no proven, reliable indicators to distinguish children whose dysphoria will desist from those in whom it will persist."[37]

Dreger explains the challenge desistance poses to the gender affirmation approach, observing,

> Most transgender activists do not want to hear that most children with gender dysphoria end up nontransgender; they want transgender to be understood as a biological, permanent, unchangeable, acceptable, natural variation. They want to welcome your child to their team and to their paradigm.[38]

33. Ristori and Steensma, "Gender Dysphoria in Childhood," 15.

34. Coleman et al., "Standards of Care," 11.

35. Temple Newhook et al., "Critical Commentary," 219.

36. Dresher and Pula, "Ethical Issues Raised," S18.

37. Dresher and Pula, "Ethical Issues Raised," S19.

38. Dreger, "Gender Identity Disorder in Childhood," 27.

The political underpinnings of the gender affirmation approach are most evident in the work of Temple Newhook et al., who question the very concept of desistance on methodological, theoretical, ethical, and interpretative grounds.[39] Temple Newhook et al. are the first gender-affirming group of professionals to challenge the longstanding desistance rate of 80 percent, suggesting that the persistence rate could be as high as twice the established standard. Zucker, himself a lifelong transgender advocate and contributing author to WPATH's *Standards of Care*, dismisses the findings of Temple Newhook et al., stating, "The 59% figure could be interpreted as implying that as many as 41% of the potential participants could have been persisters, which is an absurd inference with no empirical basis."[40] However, in spite of the high rate of desistance, proponents of gender affirmation argue for the use of GnRH agonists to treat TGNC children in order to allow for gender dysphoria symptoms to persist or desist over time. In essence, they argue that GnRH agonists buy the child time to make a decision about their gender. This suspect rationale has caused a broad spectrum of medical professionals to question the effectiveness of the gender affirmation approach.

In favor of gender affirmation, Abel assumes, "In some circumstances, the child will become comfortable with his natal gender, discontinue the GnRH, and progress through puberty as one would absent hormone interventions."[41] While this approach of buying time appears to provide a solution to gender dysphoria in theory, it fails to work in practice. Giovanardi comments, "From a psychological perspective, the main dilemma is to understand whether buying time at such a precocious age truly enables children to explore deep personal meanings, or whether it freezes youngsters in a prolonged childhood."[42] Abel later reports on a study of seventy gender-dysphoric children who were all administered GnRH agonists, noting that none of them discontinued

39. Temple Newhook et al., "Critical Commentary," 212.
40. Zucker, "Myth of Persistence," 233.
41. Abel, "Hormone Treatment of Children," S24.
42. Giovanardi, "Buying Time or Arresting Development?," 155.

puberty suppression. In spite of the fact that an overall 80 percent desistance rate exists, all seventy gender-dysphoric children who received gender affirmation therapy persisted to cross-sex hormone therapy and ultimately sexual reassignment surgery.[43] With regard to this same study, Cretella observes:

> To have 100 percent of pre-pubertal children choose cross-sex hormones suggests that the protocol itself inevitably leads the individual to identify as transgender. There is an obvious self-fulfilling nature to encouraging a young child with GD to socially impersonate the opposite sex and then institute pubertal suppression.[44]

Hruz et al. explain the self-fulfilling nature of gender affirmation as a, "looping effect, wherein the classification of people as belonging to certain 'kinds' can change how those people think of themselves and how they behave."[45] Drescher and Pula confirm the looping effect of gender affirmation, citing research that reveals for children who began the transition process, "how difficult it was for them to realize that they no longer wanted to live in the role of the other gender and make this clear to the people around them."[46] In essence, gender affirmation creates a situation where the child is either trapped or manipulated into pursuing a harmful course of permanent treatment under the guise of a temporary solution. Furthermore, Drescher and Pula assert, "No empirical evidence demonstrating that a prepubescent child who is permitted to socially transition but then desists can simply and harmlessly transition back to the natal gender."[47] Dreger confirms the findings of Drescher and Pula, citing the concerns of one gender clinician who observed that children who begin the transition process with GnRH agonists, "Cannot seem to bring themselves to tell their parents they don't want to change sex after all, after

43. Abel, "Hormone Treatment of Children," S24.
44. Cretella, "Gender Dysphoria in Children," 297.
45. Hruz et al., "Growing Pains," 26.
46. Dresher and Pula, "Ethical Issues Raised," S20.
47. Dresher and Pula, "Ethical Issues Raised," S20.

all the family has already gone through."[48] Therefore, for desisters whose symptoms of gender dysphoria are treated by the gender affirmation approach, transition back to their natal gender is not without risks, consequences, harm, injustice, and, in some cases, it is not even possible.

In summary, while there is no known cause for gender dysphoria at present, there are two opposing schools of thought with regard to etiology. One set of theories, primarily espoused by gender-affirming advocates, insists that gender dysphoria is a predetermined physical condition. A second set of theories, primarily espoused by advocates of the therapeutic model, argues that psychological or environmental factors play a prominent role in producing gender dysphoria. The evidence, particularly arising from twin studies and neuroplasticity, seems to favor environmental factors. Neuroplasticity appears to contradict brain-sex theory's assertion that gender identity is immutable, while simultaneously validating the claims of the therapeutic model. From a Christian perspective, a biblical worldview can appeal to the curse of sin (Gen 3:16–19) and the total depravity of human beings (Rom 3:10–18) in order to allow for both biological and environmental factors to play a role in the manifestation of gender dysphoria.[49] Furthermore, biblical principles indicate that parental guidance has profound influence on a child (Prov 22:6). Nevertheless, while an individual may be predisposed to certain behaviors, the shared experiences of sexual trauma, media exposure, and family dysfunction at a formative age seem to have the greatest bearing on the development of gender dysphoria and TGNC in children. And, as Hruz et al. have indicated, understanding the cause may be the key to identifying the cure.

---

48. Dreger, "Gender Identity Disorder in Childhood," 28.

49. McQuilkin and Copan, *Introduction to Biblical Ethics*, 395.

8

What are the Treatment Options for Gender-dysphoric and TGNC Children?

AT THIS POINT YOU are likely wondering, "What should I do? What are the treatment options for my gender-dysphoric or TGNC child?" The holistic treatment of gender-dysphoric and TGNC children is at the center of the ethical debate over puberty-suppressing hormones. Concerning the various conflicting approaches, Drescher and Pula stress: "There is no expert clinical consensus regarding the treatment of prepubescent children."[1] Instead, the authors maintain, "The American Psychiatric Association Task Force on the Treatment of Gender Identity outlined three differing approaches to treating gender-dysphoric children."[2] These three approaches include gender affirmation, the therapeutic model,[3] and watchful waiting.[4] With regard to these three recognized treatment options, Drescher and Pula explain:

> Due to the absence of any randomized controlled treatment outcome studies of gender-dysphoric children

1. Dresher and Pula, "Ethical Issues Raised," S17.
2. Dresher and Pula, "Ethical Issues Raised," S17.
3. Yarhouse, *Understanding Gender Dysphoria*, 105.
4. Dresher and Pula, "Ethical Issues Raised," S18.

. . . the highest level of evidence available for treatment recommendations for these children can best be characterized as expert opinion. However, there are sharp disagreements among the acknowledged experts.[5]

One approach operates under the assumption that a gender-dysphoric child is truly born with the wrong body gender. This option seeks to ease the child's distress by facilitating gender transition. A second model operates under the assumption that the child is confused. This option seeks to ease the child's distress by teaching the child to accept their physical body. A third approach argues by default that both of the former methods are inherently flawed. This option operates under the premise that the best treatment for the child is to do nothing, and to allow the child's distress to resolve naturally. No treatment option has garnered a professional scientific consensus due to lack of evidence. However, the gender affirmation approach has garnered the most public approval and political favor. Each of these approaches will be explained and critiqued, beginning with gender affirmation.

The gender affirming approach, also known as the accommodation model of treatment, is an active approach to treating gender-dysphoric and TGNC children. This approach operates under the assumption that there is nothing wrong with the child, aside from the fact that the child was born with a male brain in a female body, or vice versa.[6] Under the gender affirmation approach, society is responsible to accept the child's gender identity, support the child's gender expression, and assist the child with any social, chemical, or physical alterations that will ease that child's distress and facilitate transition. Dreger explains:

> The role of medicine, according to the accommodation model, is not to resolve [the child's] gender identity disorder, but to provide [them], when the time comes, with the hormones and surgeries [they] will need to make [their] body into what it should have always been

5. Dresher and Pula, "Ethical Issues Raised," S17.
6. Dreger, "Gender Identity Disorder in Childhood," 26.

and with the psychological support to help cope with a hostile world.[7]

Drescher and Pula describe the rationale behind gender affirming treatment as follows: "This approach presumes that an adult transgender outcome is to be expected."[8] Gender-affirmation is the only course of treatment that involves the administration of puberty-suppressing hormones. The end game for gender affirmation, from the onset, is to guide the child through gender transition.

Gender-affirming care actively supports the child's gender transition at the earliest possible age. Hruz et al. explain that this process begins when a gender-affirming therapist, "accepts, rather than challenges, the patient's self-understanding as being the opposite sex."[9] This acceptance requires the affirmation of the child's self-diagnosis at the first presentation of TGNC behaviors. Gender affirmation is immediately followed by social transition. Social transition involves both gender identity and gender expression.[10] This includes facilitating a supportive role as the child undergoes name and pronoun change, bathroom change, and proceeds to dress and act in accordance with their gender identity.[11] Social transition is followed by chemical transition, as Cretella explains: "Puberty is suppressed via GnRH agonists . . . and then finally, patients may graduate to cross-sex hormones at age 16 in preparation for sex-reassignment surgery."[12] Hruz et al. further describe the process:

> Starting at age 16, cross-sex hormones are administered while GnRH treatment continues, in order to induce something like the process of puberty that would normally occur for members of the opposite sex . . .

7. Dreger, "Gender Identity Disorder in Childhood," 27.

8. Dresher and Pula, "Ethical Issues Raised," S18.

9. Hruz et al., "Growing Pains," 4.

10. Coleman et al., "Standards of Care," 17.

11. Coleman et al., "Standards of Care," 17.

12. Cretella, "Gender Dysphoria in Children," 296.

Cross-sex hormone administration for these patients will be prescribed for the rest of their lives.[13]

The final step in the affirmation process is a series of sexual reassignment surgeries, now euphemistically referred to as corrective surgeries or the gender confirmation phase of the affirmation process. Sexual reassignment surgeries include both top and bottom procedures.[14] Top surgeries refer to cosmetic procedures intended to remove or construct secondary sexual characteristics ranging from breast implants for natal males to rhinoplasty for natal females. Proponents of gender affirmation argue that puberty suppression minimizes the need for extensive top surgeries, thereby allowing for a more convincing transition. Bottom surgeries involve the removal of the gonads, the removal of other primary sexual organs, and the surgical manufacturing of neo-genitalia. Bottom surgery can also signal the termination of GnRH agonist treatment, as Hruz et al. explain: "After the surgical removal of the gonads . . . the patients then discontinue GnRH analogue treatment, since the signaling pathway from GnRH to the pituitary gland will no longer result in the production of sex hormones."[15] However, the transgender individual must remain on cross-sex hormones for the rest of their lives.

Singal reports that, "Affirming-care has quickly become a professional imperative: Don't question who your clients are—let them tell you who they are, and accept their identity in a nurturing, encouraging manner."[16] Gender affirmation proponents insist that early intervention with puberty-suppressing hormones is in the best interest of gender-dysphoric children for six reasons. First, Dreger describes how the social benefits of gender affirmation, "allow your family to look 'normal,' taking away the unrelenting stress of having a 'different' child, [and] reducing the cruelty

13. Hruz et al., "Growing Pains," 17.

14. Dellaperute, "Church and the Transgender," 95. See my article for a detailed explanation of top and bottom surgeries.

15. Hruz et al., "Growing Pains," 17–18.

16. Singal, "Your Child Says She's Trans," 97.

you and your child encounter." [17] Second, Dreger also explains that, for persistent children, early identification and treatment will ultimately make gender transition easier. [18] Third, Temple Newhook et al. appeal to bioethics in order to support self-diagnosis, declaring, "children have their own rights to autonomy and self-determination." [19] Fourth, Abel reports how gender affirmation advocates maintain that failure to accommodate gender-dysphoric children may result in, "violent behavior, self-harm, and suicide." [20] Fifth, Kuper claims that "gender affirming medical care is considered medically necessary treatment for transgender individuals who experience physical dysphoria." [21] And finally, Kuper argues that "GnRH analogues are fully reversible intervention . . . In contrast, other aspects of gender affirming medical care are typically only partially reversible . . . or irreversible." [22]

The gender affirmation approach that advocates for the use of puberty-suppressing hormones is far from universally accepted. Yarhouse explains: "Criticisms of puberty suppression range from concerns about the effects on bone-mass development to brain development to the concern . . . about comorbid mental health issues not being resolved." [23] One primary criticism emanating from medical professionals focuses on the reliance on children to self-diagnose gender dysphoria. Drescher and Pula observe, "Increasing numbers of young children and teens are making social transitions sanctioned by families before they even come to a gender clinic." [24] This practice of self-diagnosis is a clear deviation from standard, evidence-based medical practice. Furthermore, Cretella explains that self-diagnosis is often the result of influential environmental factors, stating, "There is an increasing trend

---

17. Dreger, "Gender Identity Disorder in Childhood," 28.
18. Dreger, "Gender Identity Disorder in Childhood," 28–29.
19. Temple Newhook et al., "Critical Commentary," 219.
20. Abel, "Hormone Treatment of Children," S23.
21. Kuper, "Puberty Blocking Medications," 1.
22. Kuper, "Puberty Blocking Medications," 4.
23. Yarhouse, *Understanding Gender Dysphoria*, 108.
24. Dresher and Pula, "Ethical Issues Raised," S20.

among adolescents to self-diagnose as transgender after binges on social media."[25] Furthermore, Dreger explains that the use of GnRH agonists to treat children with gender dysphoria,

> is an off-label use. It has not been approved by the Food and Drug Administration for that purpose, and we have no good data about possible long-term negative physical or cognitive effects of using the drug this way. And some children have trouble tolerating [GnRH analogues]. It is not a magic pill.[26]

As a result, Hruz et al. argue that the administration of GnRH agonists to gender-dysphoric children constitutes, "an experiment being conducted in an uncontrolled and unsystematic manner."[27] The experimental nature of GnRH agonists is documented by Drescher and Pula, who cite Ehrensaft's trial-and-error approach as follows: "One simple rule of thumb is that if the assessment is correct, the child shows signs of getting better; if the assessment was incorrect, the child gets worse, or at least no better."[28] The experimental nature of puberty suppression directly conflicts with the evidence-based claims of WPATH and raises serious ethical concerns regarding this course of treatment for gender-dysphoric children.

Other noteworthy criticisms of gender affirmation involve both the desistance rate of gender-dysphoric children and the looping effect of the overall approach. As Singal aptly observes, "Transitioning . . . is not the answer for everyone."[29] First, Dreger asks, "What if it turns out, as it seems to with many American men who were gender dysphoric as children, that your child's dysphoria dissipates within a few years and he stops insisting he's a girl? Well, if you've followed the accommodation approach for those years, you now appear to have a daughter named Julie, in a dress, with

25. Cretella, "Gender Dysphoria in Children," 293.

26. Dreger, "Gender Identity Disorder in Childhood," 29.

27. Hruz et al., "Growing Pains," 7.

28. Dresher and Pula, "Ethical Issues Raised," S20.

29. Singal, "Your Child Says She's Trans," 94.

a penis, insisting she's a gay boy."[30] Even WPATH's *Standards of Care* reiterates Dreger's concerns regarding detransition, clearly stating, "A change back to the original gender role can be highly distressing."[31] Singal verifies this cautionary statement, documenting the painful detransition of children who were, "encouraged to rush into physical transition by clinicians operating within a framework that saw it as the only way someone . . . could experience relief."[32]

Second, Cretella counters one bioethical charge with another, observing that gender-affirming care is, "fast becoming the new treatment standard for GD in children . . . is rooted in an unscientific gender ideology, lacks an evidence base, and violates the long-standing ethical principle of 'First do no harm.'"[33] Therefore, while gender affirmation advocates aggressively defend their radical model of treatment in popular culture as the only acceptable and medically necessary course of action, two other approaches to treating TGNC children do exist. Contra Kuper, the only professionals who consider gender affirmation medically necessary for gender-dysphoric children are in fact practitioners of the gender affirmation approach, which in itself creates an ethical conflict. Those advocating most ardently for the accommodation approach are the very ones who stand to benefit financially from an increased number of TGNC children pursuing treatment. Furthermore, as Singal rightly points out, "WPATH's *Standards of Care . . .* are nonbinding."[34] This means that it is not medically necessary to follow WPATH's gender-affirming guidelines for treating TGNC children, even if the treatment is deemed medically necessary in the opinion of gender affirmation advocates such as the WPATH contributors. And finally, as Cretella reports, "Until recently, the prevailing worldview with respect to childhood GD was that it

30. Dreger, "Gender Identity Disorder in Childhood," 28.

31. Coleman et al., "Standards of Care," 17.

32. Singal, "Your Child Says She's Trans," 98.

33. Cretella, "Gender Dysphoria in Children and Suppression of Debate," 50.

34. Singal, "Your Child Says She's Trans," 99.

reflected abnormal thinking or confusion on the part of the child that may or may not be transient. Consequently, the standard approach was either watchful waiting or pursuit of family and individual psychotherapy."[35]

Like the gender-affirming method, the therapeutic model is an active approach to treating gender-dysphoric and TGNC children. This model operates under the assumption that the gender-dysphoric child is suffering from confusion over their gender identity. Drescher and Pula clarify that the goal of the therapeutic model is to align the child's gender identity with their natal gender.[36] Dreger maintains that, under the therapeutic model, both the child and their family should be treated by a mental health professional.[37] Yarhouse explains that the therapeutic model

> encourages the same-sex parent (or grandparent or mentor) to spend more time and share positive play experiences with their child while also avoiding criticisms of the child. The parents are coached to essentially ignore cross-sex typed behavior if at all possible and identify strategies to redirect the child to behaviors that reflect more that child's gender . . . Parents praise the child for any gender-appropriate activities or play.[38]

While the therapeutic model does involve behavioral modification through environmental factors, Dreger explains that there are two distinct branches of therapy. These include individual treatment and family treatment, both of which operate under the assumption that gender dysphoria, "with the right kinds of interventions . . . can be made to dissipate."[39] Finally, the therapeutic model treats the child's distress by identifying and correcting dysfunctional family dynamics and dealing with past trauma. Dreger

---

35. Cretella, "Gender Dysphoria in Children and Suppression of Debate," 51.

36. Dresher and Pula, "Ethical Issues Raised," S18.

37. Dreger, "Gender Identity Disorder in Childhood," 26.

38. Yarhouse, *Understanding Gender Dysphoria*, 103.

39. Dreger, "Gender Identity Disorder in Childhood," 26.

explains the intent of the therapeutic model to resolve gender dysphoria in a natal male as follows:

> If his mother is depressed or clingy, if his father is physically or emotionally absent, if his parents' marriage is a stressful mess, [he] is going to keep suffering from gender role confusion, and secondarily from the anger, shame, disappointment, anxiety, and guilt that his parents may exhibit in response. Although the therapeutic model does not point to a single cause of GID, it does see familial dysfunction as an aggravating factor in virtually all cases.[40]

Like the gender affirmation approach, the therapeutic model has garnered proponents and critics alike who are apt to cite the strengths and weaknesses of this approach.

While the therapeutic model does not involve invasive surgeries or chemicals, it does require time and effort on the part of both the individual and the family seeking help for the child. The greatest strength to this approach, according to Dreger, is that the child gets to keep their genitals, sexual sensation, fertility, and avoid lifelong hormone replacement by learning to identify with their natal gender.[41] However, there are three primary criticisms of the therapeutic model, all of which emanate from proponents of gender affirmation who advocate for the minority of children whose gender dysphoria persists. First, Dreger observes, "The therapeutic model implies that your family is the problem, that you all have work to do."[42] Second, Drescher and Pula relay the concern that the therapeutic model, "demean(s) the dignity of gender-variant children."[43] And finally and most seriously, advocates of gender affirmation maintain the therapeutic model constitutes harm, child abuse, and, according to WPATH's *Standards of Care*, "is no longer considered ethical."[44]

40. Dreger, "Gender Identity Disorder in Childhood," 26.
41. Dreger, "Gender Identity Disorder in Childhood," 28.
42. Dreger, "Gender Identity Disorder in Childhood," 28.
43. Dresher and Pula, "Ethical Issues Raised," S19.
44. Coleman et al., "Standards of Care," 16.

The accusation that the therapeutic model is unethical and/ or harmful to children, while unfounded, commonly surfaces in popular culture. For example, *TIME Magazine's* Fallon Fox comments on the case of Leelah Alcorn, a MtF TG teen's suicide, by calling for the incarceration of all practitioners of the therapeutic model, stating:

> In a suicide note . . . Leelah wrote when she told her mom about being transgender, her mother "reacted extremely negatively, telling me that it was a phase, that I would never truly be a girl, that God doesn't make mistakes."
> . . . While we as Americans denounce the cruelty of other countries that engage in torture . . . the cries of tortured transgender children in this country have fallen on deaf ears because of bigotry and religious beliefs that have zero place being inserted into anything resembling mental health therapy.[45]

Fox, a MtF transgender and outspoken proponent of gender affirmation, writes under the assumption that, had Leelah Alcorn's gender dysphoria been affirmed, and had Leelah been given immediate and unlimited access to GnRH agonists, cross-sex hormones, and sexual reassignment surgeries, then Leelah would not have committed suicide. Fox blames the therapeutic model and watchful waiting for Alcorn's death.

Fox's comments depicting the therapeutic model as an abusive method intended to bring about the psychological genocide of transgender youth in America are typical of the popular and carefully framed criticisms levied by gender affirmation proponents. However, an evidence-based approach contradicts Fox's assumptions. Singal reports, "The clinicians I interviewed said they rarely encounter situations in which immediate access to hormones is the difference between suicide and survival."[46] Furthermore, Cretella maintains that conflict over the therapeutic model exists even among transgender advocates, stating:

45. Fox, "Leelah Alcorn's Suicide," para. 2.
46. Singal, "Your Child Says She's Trans," 105.

Dr. Kenneth Zucker, long acknowledged as a foremost authority on gender identity issues in children, has also been a life-long advocate for gay and transgender rights. However, much to the consternation of adult transgender activists, Zucker also believes that gender-dysphoric pre-pubertal children are best served by helping them align their gender identity with their anatomic sex.[47]

Zucker's support of the therapeutic model eventually resulted in his termination from a prestigious gender clinic,[48] in spite of the fact that WPATH's own *Standards of Care,* to which Zucker contributed, requires the following course of action for gender-dysphoric and TGNC children:

> Before any physical interventions are considered for adolescents, extensive exploration of psychological, family, and social issues should be undertaken . . . The duration of this exploration may vary considerably depending on the complexity of the situation . . . Physical interventions for adolescents . . . involve the use of GnRH analogues to suppress estrogen or testosterone production and consequently delay the physical changes of puberty.[49]

Therefore, contra Fox, not only are individual therapy, family therapy, and a watchful waiting approach consistent with WPATH's own policies, but the common assertion that the denial of gender affirmation will result in self-harm is founded on pure and undocumented speculation. When gender affirmation advocates recommend immediate chemical intervention for gender-dysphoric children, they are acting in violation of their own radical standards of care.

While the gender-affirming approach and the therapeutic model offer diametrically opposing treatment methods for gender-dysphoric children, they do share two common factors. First,

47. Cretella, "Gender Dysphoria in Children and Suppression of Debate," 50.

48. Cretella, "Gender Dysphoria in Children and Suppression of Debate," 50.

49. Coleman et al., "Standards of Care," 18.

both approaches must make an assumption about the child's gender identity. They differ in the fact that gender affirmation operates under the presupposition that the child has correctly expressed their gender identity, and the therapeutic model operates under the presupposition that the child has incorrectly expressed their gender identity. Second, both methods assume that an active approach is necessary to treat gender dysphoria. Neither of these two presuppositions are present in watchful waiting, the third method for treating gender-dysphoric children.

In stark contrast to the first two treatment options, watchful waiting is a passive, alternative approach to treating gender-dysphoric and TGNC children. Gender affirmation advocates Meier and Harris succinctly describe watchful waiting as a, "'wait and see' if these behaviors desist' approach."[50] Yarhouse explains:

> "Watchful waiting" . . . or a "wait and see" approach . . . cross-gender behavior is permitted. In that way, it contrasts with psychosocial interventions to reduce cross-gender behavior and identification, as it tries to be neutral in response to such expressions. The primary difference between watchful waiting and facilitating a transition . . . is that there is not an *a priori* assumption in place that functions as a goal for the child's gender identity.[51]

The watchful waiting approach is grounded in the documented desistance rates of gender-dysphoric children and considers both the gender affirmation and therapeutic models as forms of manipulation. Watchful waiting presumes that, in most cases, the child will naturally grow to accept their natal gender without intervention. Under this method, the child is permitted some latitude in gender exploration and expression. Drescher and Pula reveal that watchful waiting remains the standard practice of some pioneering gender clinics. They explain that it involves:

---

50. Meier and Harris, "Fact Sheet," para. 4.

51. Yarhouse, *Understanding Gender Dysphoria*, 105–6.

No direct efforts to lessen gender dysphoria or gender atypical behavior. Given that GD diagnosed in childhood usually does not persist into adolescence and no reliable markers exist to predict when it will or will not persist, there is no therapeutic target with respect to gender identity outcome.[52]

Ristori and Steensma further comment on watchful waiting, stating: "Parents are encouraged to provide enough space for their child to explore their gender dysphoric feelings, while at the same time keeping all future outcomes open."[53]

The strength of the watchful waiting approach ultimately lies in its appeal to the desistance rate of gender-dysphoric children. At its core, gender dysphoria is not a physical disease, but rather a state of emotional distress that can and usually does resolve over time. Singal documents the successful resolution of gender dysphoria in a young teenage natal female whose parents, "loved and supported her . . . thanked her for telling them what she was feeling. But they stopped short of encouraging her to transition . . . [and] let her completely explore this on her own."[54] Advocates of watchful waiting argue that, if not interfered with, children will simply outgrow the distress associated with gender dysphoria and learn to accept their natal gender.

There are two primary criticisms of the watchful waiting approach, both of which emanate from proponents of the gender affirmation approach. First, the passive nature of this method is questioned on a pragmatic level. Kuvalanka et al. explain:

> If family members are waiting for a child to decide upon gender pronouns, those family members may experience a feeling of being "in limbo" . . . Labels to define their relationships may not exist, leaving them to grapple with: If you are not my son or daughter, sister or brother, niece or nephew, then who are you to me? Further, parents may struggle to advocate for children with nonbinary gender

52. Dresher and Pula, "Ethical Issues Raised," S18.
53. Ristori and Steensma, "Gender Dysphoria in Childhood," 17.
54. Singal, "Your Child Says She's Trans," 90.

identities in schools if neither the girls nor boys bathroom quite fits, or when children are required to "line up," use gym locker rooms, or participate in sports according to binary gender groupings. Children with nonbinary trans identities "may challenge family members and others to critically examine the embedded nature of gender binaries in human societies" . . . in ways that acceptance of a binary trans child's identity may not.[55]

Second, Kuper summarizes the position most gender affirmation advocates take concerning watchful waiting as follows: "In light of the irreversible changes that occur during puberty, specialists who work with transgender adolescents emphasize that 'wait and see' approaches are not neutral responses to persistent gender dysphoria."[56] Winters et al. emphasize the need to act immediately with gender affirmation by condemning watchful waiting as follows:

> Most importantly, it dismisses children's profound internal experiences of their own gender. Though labelled as "watchful waiting and carefully observing," such discouragement of congruent gender expression and authentic participation in childhood life experience is not a neutral clinical choice. In our experience, childhood closets can have lifelong consequences.[57]

However, the gender-affirming assumptions of Winters et al. do stand in stark contrast to WPATH's recommendations regarding extensive exploration of psychological, family, and social issues prior to pursuing puberty suppression.[58]

After examining three profoundly different treatment options, parents, medical professionals, and ministers are faced with a serious, life-altering ethical dilemma when deciding how to help gender-dysphoric and TGNC children resolve their distress. At present, the culturally dominant view is to implement

55. Kuvalanka et al., "Trans and Gender-nonconforming Children," 897.

56. Kuper, "Puberty Blocking Medications," 8.

57. Winters et al., "Learning to Listen," 248.

58. Coleman et al., "Standards of Care," 18.

gender affirmation, which facilitates gender transition at a young age, beginning with puberty suppression. In spite of the fact that no medical consensus exists, gender affirmation advocates have garnered so much popular support that its practitioners are now seeking to prohibit all other treatment options by portraying the therapeutic model as an active form child abuse and watchful waiting as a passive form of neglect. In contrast to gender affirmation, the therapeutic model, which has until recently been the standard approach to treating gender dysphoria, seeks to help the TGNC child accept their natal gender by addressing environmental factors that aggravate feelings of distress in gender-dysphoric children. Finally, a third method, while passive in nature, is still radical in its approach. Watchful waiting maintains that the best treatment option for gender dysphoria is to do nothing to affirm or reprove the child, and instead allow the child to pass through a period gender nonconformity without interference. Ironically, all three methods simultaneously appeal to the same elements of bioethical principlism in order to justify their respective positions.

9

Are Puberty-suppressing Hormones Unethical for Gender-dysphoric Children?

As a parent, medical care provider, or ministry professional, you now have to choose between gender affirmation, the therapeutic model, and watchful waiting. Which one is the right choice for treating gender dysphoria in children? If you choose gender affirmation, your child will begin treatment with GnRH agonists. However, you must answer the question: "Is puberty suppression an ethical course of treatment for gender-dysphoric children?" Cretella aptly maintains, "the debate over how to treat children with GD is primarily an ethical dispute."[1] Therefore, after clarifying the terminology, biology, etiology, and arguments for and against treating gender-dysphoric children with synthetic puberty-suppressing hormones, this contemporary practice can now be fairly evaluated by applying biomedical ethics.

de S. Cameron defines bioethics as, "The supremely interdisciplinary discipline [which] stands at the confluence of biomedical sciences, law, philosophy, theology, and of course, ethics itself."[2] The importance of biomedical ethics lies in the fact that, like any

1. Cretella, "Gender Dysphoria in Children," 287.
2. de S. Cameron, "Bioethics," 323.

other treatment in secular culture, moral justification for the decision to administer puberty-suppressing hormones under the auspices of gender affirmation is determined by whether or not it meets the four recognized criteria of ethical principlism.[3] The industry standard for bioethical norms is explained by Beauchamp and Childress as a set of, "pivotal moral principles . . . [that] function as an analytical framework of general norms derived from the common morality that form a suitable starting point for biomedical ethics."[4] However, from an evangelical perspective, it can also be demonstrated that the four philosophical pillars that guide biomedical ethics are also elements of common grace and, when applied in a consistent manner, constitute biblical principles.[5]

The four pillars of medical bioethics are nonmaleficence, beneficence, justice, and respect for autonomy.[6] Although some contemporary debate occurs regarding which principle takes precedence over the others in matters of apparent ethical conflict, historically nonmaleficence and beneficence have long been considered the medical practitioner's primary responsibilities, with nonmaleficence positioned as first among equals. Beauchamp and Childress explain: "Nonmaleficence and beneficence have played a central role in the history of medical ethics. By contrast, respect for autonomy and justice were neglected in traditional medical ethics and have risen to prominence only recently."[7]

The principle of nonmaleficence, often considered the preeminent principle of the Hippocratic Oath, is, "First do no harm."[8] This moral standard identifies any activity or procedure that causes harm to another as unethical. The principle of nonmaleficence is consistent with biblical teaching, which instructs that, "Love does no harm to a neighbor. Therefore love is the fulfillment of the law"

---

3. Abel, "Hormone Treatment of Children," S25.

4. Beauchamp and Childress, *Principles of Biomedical Ethics*, 13.

5. de S. Cameron, "Bioethics," 324.

6. Beauchamp and Childress, *Principles of Biomedical Ethics*, 13.

7. Beauchamp and Childress, *Principles of Biomedical Ethics*, 13.

8. Beauchamp and Childress, *Principles of Biomedical Ethics*, 150.

(Rom 13:10 NIV).[9] Second, the principle of beneficence maintains that there exists, "a moral obligation to act for the benefit of others."[10] Scripture also supports the principle of beneficence, as is evident in the royal law (Jas 2:8) and in the account of the good Samaritan.[11] The two principles of nonmaleficence and beneficence have traditionally guided all biomedical procedures from ancient times. As de S. Cameron explains, "the readiness with which Christians embraced Hippocratic medicine, and even its plainly pagan oath, underlies its fundamental congruence with a Christian agenda for medical values."[12]

The third principle of biomedical ethics is justice, which Beauchamp and Childress define as follows: "Distributive justice refers to fair, equitable, and appropriate distribution of benefits and burdens."[13] Justice ensures the fair treatment of all patients regardless of race, age, gender, vulnerability, or financial factors. Concerning its spiritual significance, Christ himself identifies justice as one of the, "more important matters of the law" (Matt 23:23 NIV). The final pillar of bioethics is respect for autonomy. As Beauchamp and Childress explain, "At a minimum, respect for autonomy encompasses self-rule that is free from both controlling interference by others and limitations that prevent meaningful choice."[14] Here, Beauchamp and Childress do not advocate for unrestrained autonomy, but instead proceed to qualify this ethical principle with two mitigating factors. First, the authors state, "we do not hold, as some of our critics have suggested, that the principle of respect for autonomy always has priority over all other moral considerations."[15] Second, Beauchamp and Childress stress that respect for autonomy, like the first three pillars, is,

---

9. All quotations will be cited from the NIV unless otherwise specified.

10. Beauchamp and Childress, *Principles of Biomedical Ethics*, 203.

11. Beauchamp and Childress, *Principles of Biomedical Ethics*, 203.

12. de S. Cameron, "Bioethics," 327.

13. Beauchamp and Childress, *Principles of Biomedical Ethics*, 250.

14. Beauchamp and Childress, *Principles of Biomedical Ethics*, 101.

15. Beauchamp and Childress, *Principles of Biomedical Ethics*, 101.

"subject to specification."[16] Beauchamp and Childress ultimately modify autonomy with the three factors of acting intentionally, understanding the process, and performing an action that is free from controlling influences.[17] Finally, like nonmaleficence, beneficence, and justice, modified autonomy is a biblically supported principle. Scripture states: "You, my brothers and sisters, were called to be free. But do not use your freedom to indulge the flesh; rather, serve one another humbly in love" (Gal 5:13).

The use of puberty-suppressing hormones on gender-dysphoric children must satisfy these four established principles in order to be considered an ethical treatment option. At times, an apparent conflict does exist. The primary arguments in favor of treating gender-dysphoric children with puberty-suppressing hormones appeal to the principle of autonomy. The primary arguments against treating gender-dysphoric children puberty-suppressing hormones often appeal to the principles of nonmaleficence and beneficence. Therefore, we will proceed to evaluate the ethical justification for the use of puberty-suppressing hormones to treat gender-dysphoric and TGNC children with an emphasis on nonmaleficence and autonomy in an attempt to resolve this conflict.

The first question that parents, medical providers, and ministry professionals must ask when seeking treatment for gender-dysphoric and TGNC children is: "Will this approach harm the child?" As examined in the biochemical evaluation of puberty, the administration of puberty-suppressing hormones does interfere with the holistic growth process of the human being by preventing the normal development of primary and secondary sexual characteristics. This interruption is known to arrest bone growth, interfere with brain maturation, and ultimately result in infertility. Other adverse side effects will likely emerge over time as the first generation of gender-dysphoric children who received GnRH agonists continues to age. Even WPATH's *Standards of Care* admits "there are concerns about negative physical side effects of GnRH

16. Beauchamp and Childress, *Principles of Biomedical Ethics*, 19.
17. Beauchamp and Childress, *Principles of Biomedical Ethics*, 104.

analogue use."[18] However, in spite of these known adverse effects and suspected concerns, Jamie Dean reports, "In 2016 the Obama administration demanded most physicians facilitate gender transitions for any child referred by a mental health professional, even if the doctor thought the process harmful to children."[19] This edict essentially voids the first principle of bioethics. Furthermore, children who begin puberty suppression must progress to cross-sex hormones in order to continue the transition process. As noted earlier, gender-affirming clinicians are disregarding WPATH's *Standards of Care* and prescribing cross-sex hormones to children at increasingly younger ages. Concerning cross-sex hormones, Abel confesses:

> This principle [nonmaleficence] offers the strongest ethical argument against cross-sex hormone treatment because the long-term effects of this therapy are not well known; only a single patient has been the subject of long-term follow-up. Additionally, cross-sex therapy has the known side effect of rendering most patients sterile.[20]

Therefore, nonmaleficence presents a moral stumbling block for advocates of gender affirmation due to the fact that GnRH agonists do harm to gender-dysphoric children.

Proponents of gender affirmation attempt to circumvent the principle of nonmaleficence by one of two avenues. First, Abel argues that GnRH agonists, "Have largely been considered free of long-term harm; this assertion is supported by many generations of follow-up studies with the large population of individuals prescribed such drugs for precocious puberty."[21] However, careful examination of Abel's explanation reveals that gender affirmation advocates must employ sleight-of-hand with scientific data in order to make such a sweeping assertion. Arguing that GnRH agonists offer a safe and effective treatment for gender dysphoria

18. Coleman et al., "Standards of Care," 20.
19. Dean, "Suffer the Children," para. 12.
20. Abel, "Hormone Treatment of Children," S25.
21. Abel, "Hormone Treatment of Children," S25.

based on their success with treating precocious puberty is akin to arguing for the use of chemotherapy to treat ADHD due to its effectiveness on cancer. GnRH agonists, when administered to children with the biological disorder of precocious puberty, normalize an irregular maturation process. The synthetic hormones are then discontinued at the beginning of Tanner Stage II. In contrast, GnRH agonists are administered to gender-dysphoric children who exhibit emotional distress over their natal gender beginning at Tanner Stage II. The intent of this treatment is to interrupt the normal maturation process. Hormone therapy for gender-dysphoric children then continues through Tanner Stage V. This means that gender-dysphoric children who are prescribed GnRH agonists are given the synthetic hormones at a significantly older age than children with precocious puberty, remain on the synthetic hormones for a significantly longer period of time, and take the synthetic hormones at a completely different stage of maturation and for a completely different purpose. Furthermore, GnRH agonists were first synthesized in 1971 and first administered to children with precocious puberty a decade later. No empirical data on the effects of GnRH agonists for the treatment of gender dysphoria even existed until 2011, when Cohen-Kettenis reported on a single case study that began in 1998.[22] Even WPATH's own *Standards of Care* admits to the lack of scientific evidence for GnRH use, stating "the long term effects can only be determined when the earliest treated patients reach the appropriate age."[23] Therefore, it can be demonstrated that even the staunchest advocates of gender affirmation like WPATH must admit that no scientific evidence base exists to support the theory that puberty suppression is a harmless, reversible, or even effective treatment option for gender-dysphoric children. Any appeals to the safety or effectiveness of treating gender-dysphoric children with GnRH agonists based on "generations of follow-up studies" are simply not evidence-based. Instead, they are fabricated by manipulating the data derived from the treatment of children with precocious puberty. This data

22. Cohen-Kettenis et al., "Puberty Suppression," 843.
23. Coleman et al., "Standards of Care," 20.

manipulation not only causes harm to children while directly benefiting advocates of gender affirmation, but it also directly impacts other bioethical principles, since understanding is one of the three specifications for autonomy.[24] As a result, Cretella aptly concludes, "This protocol is rooted in an unscientific gender ideology, lacks an evidence base, and violates the long-standing ethical principle of 'First do no harm.'"[25]

Hann et al. take a different approach to denying the charge of nonmaleficence, arguing, "Nonmaleficence implies a commitment to medical competence by minimizing harm to patients. In healthcare, harm is seen in barriers to access care, perpetuation of stigma and discrimination, and omission of risks."[26] Newhook et al. echo these concerns, insisting that failure to provide access to puberty-suppressing hormones constitutes harm to gender-dysphoric children.[27] However, by appealing to access to healthcare under the framework of nonmaleficence, gender affirmation proponents either misunderstand, misrepresent, or attempt to redefine the ethical principle of harm with the new language of gender.[28] Concerning nonmaleficence, Beauchamp and Childress clearly explain:

> From the principle that we should avoid causing harm to persons, there is no direct step to the conclusion that a positive obligation exists to provide benefits such as health care and various forms of assistance . . . Obligations to provide positive benefits are the territory of beneficence and justice.[29]

24. Beauchamp and Childress, *Principles of Biomedical Ethics*, 131.

25. Cretella, "Gender Dysphoria in Children and Suppression of Debate," 50.

26. Hann et al., "Bioethics in Practice," 144.

27. Temple Newhook et al., "Critical Commentary," 219.

28. Zucker, "Myth of Persistence," 240. Zucker describes Temple Newhook et al.'s conclusion as follows: "This is a gross oversimplification, an oversimplification that Temple Newhook et al. require in order to assimilate their interpretation of the data into their theoretical/ethical argumentation" (240).

29. Beauchamp and Childress, *Principles of Biomedical Ethics*, 192–93.

Therefore, nonmaleficence occurs when medical intervention directly causes harm. Harm resulting from refusing to provide treatment may be considered under an appeal to justice or beneficence, but not nonmaleficence. Notwithstanding, even the assertion that withholding puberty suppression harms gender-dysphoric children is yet another undocumented assumption by advocates of gender affirmation. As previously explained, no scientific evidence exists to prove that failing to provide GnRH agonists to a gender-dysphoric or TGNC child will harm the child in any way. On the contrary, due to the harm directly caused by puberty suppression, even Drescher and Pula warn, "a cautious approach is warranted."[30] Finally, considering the 80 percent desistance rate, if the administration of GnRH agonists to gender-dysphoric children becomes standard medical practice, then four out of five children will be needlessly treated with synthetic hormones that will unnecessarily alter their bodies and accentuate their distress. As a result of this evidence, the answer to the question of whether or not puberty-suppressing hormones will harm a gender-dysphoric child is yes. However, this is not the only question that needs to be asked.

The next question that parents, medical providers, and ministry professionals must ask when considering puberty suppression for gender-dysphoric and TGNC children is: "Is the child capable of making autonomous medical decisions?" Advocates of the gender affirmation approach champion the argument that gender-dysphoric children have a right to access puberty-suppressing hormones under the principle of autonomy. This appeal to autonomy creates an apparent ethical conflict with nonmaleficence. In order to resolve this conflict, gender affirmation proponents give precedence to autonomy. For example, Abel explains, "Respect for autonomy is the strongest factor supporting progressive hormone treatments."[31] Furthermore, Hann et al. insist: "Transgender patients have the right to have their self-identification respected . . . In addition, transgender patients have the right to make healthcare

30. Dresher and Pula, "Ethical Issues Raised," S19.

31. Abel, "Hormone Treatment of Children," S25.

decisions collaboratively with their providers under the principle of informed consent."[32] Temple-Newhook et al. also argue that a child's autonomy ought to be prioritized over all other ethical considerations.[33] However, this assertion is far from universally accepted. Even WPATH's *Standards of Care* recognizes that, "Ideally, treatment decisions should be made among the adolescent, the family, and the treatment team."[34] So, does the principle of autonomy mandate that the decisions of the family and treatment team must always affirm the self-diagnosis and decisions of the gender-dysphoric or TGNC child in every situation?

Autonomy provides neither a preeminent ethical factor nor a license for unrestricted practice in bioethics. Drescher and Pula explain that children are not considered autonomous because "they are deemed developmentally immature and unable to fully understand the risks and benefits of medical decision-making."[35] Abel concurs with Drescher and Pula, stating:

> Children are generally unable to provide autonomous, independent informed consent for medical treatments. This long-standing tenant of pediatric care protects children who often do not possess fully developed cognitive decision-making capacity by preventing rash, permanent, and potentially regrettable medical decisions . . . Until a youth reaches the age of majority, the medical decision-making process generally includes permission from parents or guardians and informed assent from the patient to the degree appropriate . . . the likelihood is too high that the child would be unable to comprehend the scope of a decision that carries significant, permanent consequences.[36]

Cretella offers scientific insight into why children are not deemed autonomous, stating, "Neuroscience clearly documents

32. Hann et al., "Bioethics in Practice," 144.
33. Temple Newhook et al., "Critical Commentary," 221.
34. Coleman et al., "Standards of Care," 20.
35. Dresher and Pula, "Ethical Issues Raised," S19.
36. Abel, "Hormone Treatment of Children," S23.

that the adolescent brain is cognitively immature and lacks an adult capacity for risk assessment."[37] Finally, Singal also reports, "The developing teenage brain . . . is more susceptible to peer influence, more impulsive, and less adept at weighing long-term outcomes and consequences than fully developed adult brains."[38] Therefore, although children and adolescents may truly experience distress associated with gender dysphoria, the presence of distress, a self-diagnosis, or even a diagnosis by a gender affirmation specialist does not ethically qualify the child for puberty suppression under the principle of modified autonomy. In order for an action to be autonomous, specification requires that the action must not only be free from influencing factors, but its implications must be generally understood by the patient. Gender-dysphoric children do not meet either of these established criteria for the actual biomedical ethic of autonomy. Therefore, the answer to the question of whether or not a child should be permitted to pursue puberty suppression based on a self-diagnosis of gender dysphoria under an appeal to autonomy is no. Parents, medical providers, and ministry professionals must serve as gatekeepers and act in the best interests of the child by protecting gender-dysphoric and TGNC children from harm and future regret.

The third question that parents, medical practitioners, and ministry professionals must ask when considering synthetic hormone treatment for gender-dysphoric and TGNC children is: "Am I morally obligated to provide this course of treatment?"[39] Abel explains that the principle of beneficence "obligates physicians to help their patients."[40] On these grounds, gender affirmation advocates like Hann et al. argue, "Beneficence implies addressing barriers to care and healthcare disparities on both the population and individual level. This approach to healthcare for all patients

37. Cretella, "Gender Dysphoria in Children and Suppression of Debate," 52.

38. Singal, "Your Child Says She's Trans," 106.

39. Beauchamp and Childress, *Principles of Biomedical Ethics*, 203.

40. Abel, "Hormone Treatment of Children," S26.

should be affirmative, understanding, and nonjudgmental."[41] With this definition, Hann et al. appeal to beneficence as a means of preventing parents or medical professionals from serving as gate-keepers and questioning the self-diagnosis of gender-dysphoric children. Instead of seeking the best interest of the child, the prevailing influence of autonomy on beneficence seeks to create a system of entitlement that allows gender affirmation advocates to discard the essential nature of paternalism. The attack on paternalism is evident in the legal battle over Ohio's Parents' Rights Bill.[42]

Paternalism is a form of gatekeeping that falls under the bio-ethical category of beneficence. For example, if a drug addict were to demand a prescription for opioids by appealing to autonomy, "I want the pills because I think I need them," and beneficence, "Since it is within your power to give me the pills, you must honor my wishes," most doctors would choose to deny the request based on paternalism. Beauchamp and Childress explain:

> We define "paternalism" as the intentional overriding of one person's preferences or actions by another person, where the person who is overriding justifies this action by appeal to the goal of benefiting or of preventing or mitigating harm to the person whose preferences or actions are overridden.[43]

However, regarding gender dysphoria, *Time Magazine's* Jennifer Calfas explains that opponents of the Parents' Rights Bill, comprised primarily of gender affirmation and LGBTQ activists, legally challenged whether parents have a right to decide what is in the best interest of their own children.[44] At its core, paternalism maintains that is the responsibility of parents, with aid from medical practitioners and ministry professionals, to advise against or even override harmful or medically unnecessary procedures in the name of beneficence, even if the child insists. For, if comorbid factors such as sexual trauma, autism, or family dysfunction are

---

41. Hann et al., "Bioethics in Practice," 144.
42. Calfas, "Ohio Bill."
43. Beauchamp and Childress, *Principles of Biomedical Ethics*, 215.
44. Calfas, "Ohio Bill."

an underlying cause of gender dysphoria, as the evidence seems to suggest, then GnRH agonists will not contribute to the health, well-being, or benefit of the child. Furthermore, regarding gender affirmation appeals to beneficence, Abel explains, "a finding of a high prevalence of desistance detracts from the argument for beneficence."[45] Finally, the administration of GnRH agonists is not a medical necessity, but instead represents a very recent and highly controversial opinion by a group of individuals who stand to benefit financially from the child's decision to transition. Other courses of treatment, including therapy and watchful waiting, do exist. Therefore, the answer to the question of whether parents and medical providers are obligated to provide puberty-suppressing hormones to gender-dysphoric children is no.

The final question that parents, medical providers, and ministry professionals must ask when considering puberty suppression for gender-dysphoric and TGNC children is: "Is this a fair, equitable, and appropriate distribution of benefits and burdens?"[46] This is a question that insurance companies, government programs, and society in general must also consider in light of the costs associated with GnRH agonists. Hann et al. rightly maintain that "transgender patients are equally entitled to a fair distribution of healthcare resources."[47] However, the issue at stake is not whether gender-dysphoric or TGNC children should be denied basic medical care. The issue concerning what constitutes fair and equitable treatment is at the center of this debate. In short, should society assume responsibility for providing GnRH agonists to all gender-dysphoric and TGNC children? Gender-affirming advocates such as Hann et al. insist that government agencies and insurance companies are in fact responsible for hormone therapy and all transition-related surgeries.[48] However, these procedures come at a great expense that will place unnecessary and unjust stress on an already overburdened system.

45. Abel, "Hormone Treatment of Children," S26.

46. Beauchamp and Childress, *Principles of Biomedical Ethics*, 250.

47. Hann et al., "Bioethics in Practice," 144.

48. Hann et al., "Bioethics in Practice," 145.

Stevens et al. explain that "GnRH agonist pharmacotherapy can cost thousands of dollars per month."[49] Stevens proceeds to cite Dr. Norman Spack, a leading endocrinologist at Boston's Children's Hospital, indicating that the cost of the most commonly prescribed puberty-suppressing hormone therapy exceeds $2,000 per month per child.[50] Therefore, if a gender-dysphoric child were to begin treatment with GnRH agonists at a typical age, say nine years old, and then progress to cross-sex hormones at age sixteen, and finally proceed to surgical removal of the gonads at age eighteen, this process would require nine years of treatment with puberty-suppressing hormones. These nine years represent the legal minimum under the current gender affirmation approach, although some of its most radical adherents have begun to disregard WPATH's *Standards of Care* and administer cross-sex hormones before age sixteen and pursue bottom surgery before the age of majority.[51] Furthermore, some gender-dysphoric and TGNC individuals do not pursue bottom surgery until much later in life, if at all, thereby extending the use of puberty suppressors indefinitely. However, if the gender-dysphoric child were to cease GnRH agonists after nine years, setting all known and unknown physical and psychological side effects aside, the cost alone for puberty suppression at present would exceed $216,000 per child. Furthermore, if Singal's earlier figure of 150,000 gender-dysphoric children at present in the US is correct, then it would cost in excess of $75 billion to provide puberty suppression for those children currently experiencing gender dysphoria.

While the costs of GnRH agonists can seem prohibitive when so many other devastating childhood illnesses and disorders like autism, cancer, cystic fibrosis, diabetes, meningitis, etc. plague our planet, their use can be justified if they are determined to be medically necessary to save the life of a child. Gender affirmation proponents Stevens et al. explain why puberty suppression comes at such a great expense:

49. Stevens et al., "Insurance Coverage," 1029.

50. Stevens et al., "Insurance Coverage," 1029.

51. Coleman et al., "Standards of Care," 20–21.

The higher cost of pharmaceuticals approved for use in youth may be related to the increased complexity and cost of clinical trials in children, the high risk of conducting these trials, the low expectation of return on this investment, and the designation of a new drug that extends patent exclusivity in exchange for trials in children.[52]

Furthermore, the $216,000 figure does not include the significant medical fees associated with cross-sex hormones, transition surgeries, or any additional transgender-related procedures like regular visits to pediatric endocrinologists or gender affirmation therapists who, once again, stand to benefit directly from the very procedures they promote.[53] The figure is solely restricted to covering the fees associated with puberty-suppressing hormones.

The implications of this financial burden on the ethical principle of justice are serious. For if, as gender affirmation advocates acknowledge, at least four out of five gender-dysphoric children desist without the aid of puberty suppression, and if, as gender affirmation proponents also admit, it is impossible to distinguish the children that will desist from the ones that may persist, then for every five gender-dysphoric children who are treated with GnRH agonists, nearly $1,000,000 of medical funding will be spent unnecessarily and unjustly on a condition that would have otherwise been resolved without any medical intervention. Four out of five children treated with GnRH agonists under the gender affirmation approach will either desist, or they will continue the transition process when they would have otherwise desisted due to the looping effect of gender affirmation. Therefore, the answer to the question of whether or not providing puberty-suppressing hormones to gender-dysphoric and TGNC children constitutes a just distribution of benefits and burdens is no. Puberty-suppressing hormones do not satisfy the ethical principles of nonmaleficence, autonomy, beneficence, or justice, and therefore constitute unethical treatment of gender-dysphoric and TGNC children.

52. Stevens et al., "Insurance Coverage," 1029.
53. Coleman et al., "Standards of Care," 20.

10

Is there a Biblical Alternative
for Treating Gender Dysphoria?

YOU ARE THE PARENT. You suspect there is something seriously wrong with your child. And now you know that puberty suppression provides neither an ethical nor effective solution for your child's emotional distress. But you still do not know where to turn in order to help your child. Should you seek therapy? Are you comfortable with watchful waiting? Is there anything you can do at present to help your child? This concluding section contains a theological synthesis of Scripture, science, psychology, ethics, testimonials, and practical advice that can help parents guide their child through a tumultuous period of gender dysphoria. It begins with a testimonial.

Once upon a time, there was a man who had a severely distressed son. His child's distress manifested early as mutism, and it progressed to horrific self-destructive behavior as the child reached adolescence. The man tried every means at his disposal to help his child, but nothing seemed to work. Over time, his son only grew worse. However, as sick and confused as his son became, the father held fast to three things. First, he refused to give up on his son. Instead, he was determined to love his son unconditionally, and, as a result, he continued to pursue active measures to help his child. Second, the father did not affirm his son's behavior, even though it would have been tolerated by others in his culture. And finally, the man was willing to turn to Christ's followers for help.

I wish I could report that this father's first attempt at a faith-based approach to helping his child was successful. Unfortunately, like many others, such was not the case for this man. The father's first experience with a Christian approach to resolving his son's distress was overwhelmingly negative and left him distraught. Nonetheless, he remained resolute, even though his initial disappointment caused him to question his faith. However, in time, his perseverance was rewarded. His son eventually came to Christ and was delivered from his distress. This father leaves behind a legacy of patience, persistence, and prayer for other scared and confused parents to apply when attempting to minister to their distressed children.

Although the identities of father and son remain anonymous, their story is true, and their account is recorded in Mark 9:14–29. Sharing this story is not an attempt to correlate demon possession with gender dysphoria. Instead, it provides practical biblical principles that all struggling parents can glean and apply when seeking to help their confused and hurting children. The first principle, and the one emphasized in this account and missing in gender affirmation, the therapeutic model, and watchful waiting, is prayer (Mark 9:29).

Powerful, effective prayer is essential for parents seeking to help their children resolve gender dysphoria (Jas 5:16). This is an active measure that conflicts with the "do nothing" approach of watchful waiting. The prayer life of a parent whose child is suffering from gender dysphoria should not only include praying for your child, but it also involves praying with your child. Like any crisis, this is an opportunity to teach your child to share their depression, confusion, and anxieties with the Lord, knowing that God cares for them (1 Pet 5:7). First, encourage your child to be honest with God. After all, Christ understands human struggles and weaknesses better than anyone else (Heb 2:18). Second, remind your child that, even though the situation may seem bleak, God is able to do immeasurably more than all we ask or imagine (Eph 3:20). Third, do not neglect confessing your own sins and struggles when you pray with your child (Jas 5:16), and encourage, but do not require, your child to confess their sin as well (1 John 1:9). Be discrete and appropriate, but lead by example. Fourth, be sure to thank God for your child every time you pray, regardless of whether you prayers are private or corporate (Phil 1:3–4). Your gender-dysphoric child is still God's gift to you (Ps 127:3), and they need to be secure in your love for them. Finally, when you pray in private, ask the Lord to search you, and test you, and see if there is any sinful behavior that you need to change (Ps 139:23–24). And then, make those changes in your life.

The second principle is that before you can treat the speck of gender dysphoria in your child's life, you may need to remove some immoral planks in your own life (Matt 7:3–5). Herein lies the strength of the therapeutic model. Known sinful behavior in your life, your home, your marriage, or your family is likely contributing to your child's gender dysphoria. You cannot expect to help your child to change if you are unwilling to change first. Consider the prayer of the desperate father, "Help *me* overcome *my* unbelief" (Mark 9:24). For example, if there is adultery, pornography, sexual sin, or substance abuse in your life, then you need to repent and make some necessary changes, because these parental sins are likely aggravating your child's gender identity struggles. Furthermore, if your marriage is in crisis, you need to work to resolve your relationship with your spouse. And, if you are already divorced, do not use your separation as an excuse to throw in the towel. Instead, as much as depends on you, live at peace with everyone (Rom 12:18), including your ex-spouse. This means forgive, reconcile if possible, and do your part to reduce the animosity and stress in your home. As a general rule, increased conflict between parents will produce more distress in the life of any child. Resolving family conflict is crucial to resolving gender dysphoria. Also, if your approach to parenting can best be described as extremely detached or extremely overbearing, you need to learn to adjust your behavior for the well-being of your child. Change starts with you, the parent, but it does not end with you.

Third, closely examine your child's relationships, because bad company corrupts good character every time (1 Cor 15:33). As a parent, the most dangerous position you can assume at this junction is one of willful ignorance. Therefore, after taking a long, hard look at your own life, you need to closely examine every person of influence in your child's life, including their friends, relatives, babysitters, teachers, counselors, coaches, and even pastors. Be suspicious of anyone your child is overly attached to or extremely anxious around. You also need to have regular conversations with your child about appropriate and inappropriate touch. Sadly, sexual assault is a common denominator shared by many children and adolescents who experience gender dysphoria. Furthermore, an influential adult activist does not need to molest a child in order to push gender ideology onto an impressionable young mind. As a parent, there is a time to enact paternalism and end unhealthy relationships for the well-being of your child. And, if a crime has been committed, seek justice for the offender and healing for the survivor. Remember, just as a child cannot consent to medical procedures, they cannot consent to sexual activity, especially if that activity involves coercion by someone significantly older. The child is the victim in these situations, and they need compassion and grace from their parents, not judgment.

Fourth, remove any damaging influences from your child, and remove your child from any dangerous environments. This is another active, radical step that needs to be taken in order to resolve gender dysphoria. If social media is causing your child to stumble, as it does in many instances, then pluck it out of your child's life (Mark 9:47). Media influence has a profound effect on impressionable young minds, and the internet is saturated with transgender activism. Hidden algorithms in websites and search engines steer unsuspecting children toward gender affirming sites. While removing access, restricting content, and monitoring activity are three essentials for every parent of a digital-age child, these steps are even more crucial for parents of children struggling with gender dysphoria. For example, Singal documents how a modified watchful waiting approach that was implemented by the parents of a TGNC natal female helped their daughter "Claire" successfully navigate through a period of gender dysphoria. Claire's dysphoria was directly influenced by media events, and by restricting access to online outlets, Claire's distress eventually desisted.[1] Furthermore, if a public school environment is causing your child to stumble due to student or adult activism, then take your child out. This, too, is a function of paternalism. In this case, it would be better to homeschool or pay for a private Christian school with shared values than to allow your child to remain under the constant pressure and influence of gender affirmation advocates.

Fifth, you should encourage your child to keep a journal of their thoughts and feelings. Your child should read this journal with you at regular intervals and reflect on their progress. This technique was also very helpful in the life of Claire.[2] Journaling should be done with the understanding that you and your child are on a journey to discover the truth, not affirm their self-diagnosis. So do not be discouraged, because God's word is truth (John 17:17). Therefore it is also appropriate to assign your child a portion of Scripture to read, reflect on, and respond to in their journal along with their thoughts and feelings. Two healthy places to begin are Genesis 1–3 and the Gospel of Mark. And remember, like all journeys, there will be sunny days, and there will be storms. Resist the urge to declare your child cured after a week of apparent desistance, and do not overreact to their persistent TGNC claims. Even the gender affirmation advocates of WPATH require six to twelve months of insistent, persistent, and consistent behavior before a diagnosis of gender dysphoria can technically be made by their own radical standards. So learn a lesson from the Mark 9 father and be patient and persistent. Herein lies the strength of watchful waiting. While there is no set time limit to resolving gender dysphoria, most distress does desist over time.

1. Singal, "Your Child Says She's Trans," 90.
2. Singal, "Your Child Says She's Trans," 91.

Sixth, parents of gender-dysphoric children must turn to Christ, like the father in Mark 9, and carefully enlist other trusted believers to help them with their child. This will not be easy for the parents, the child, or church, since there is often a stigma associated with gender dysphoria and TGNC. However, Christ did not call his followers to easy living (Mark 8:34). A church family can and should bathe the situation in prayer. A church can provide support and accountability for the parents of gender-dysphoric children who need to enact changes in their own lives. A church can also provide guidance and mentoring for the child (Prov 11:14). A healthy relationship with an understanding individual of the same natal gender as the child can be extremely helpful in resolving gender dysphoria. Furthermore, a church can and must provide compassion for struggling children (Mark 10:14). The distress associated with gender dysphoria is real, and shame and exclusion are not effective treatment options. Ostracizing the child or family is just as damaging as affirming the child, and woe to that person who causes a child to stumble (Mark 9:42). If Christ's own disciples could welcome a demon-possessed child into their company, then surely the contemporary evangelical church can find a place for children struggling with gender dysphoria. Church leadership can also provide guidance concerning professional therapeutic options that avoid gender affirmation, particularly in cases of self-harm or where comorbid factors such as autism or sexual trauma are contributing to gender dysphoria. Finally, the goal of the church should be the salvation and spiritual growth of the child, since Christ came, lived, died, and rose again to redeem and restore the sick and hurting (Mark 2:17).

Seventh, with gentleness and respect, parents need to hold the line on a fixed, biblical gender binary of male and female. This approach will require parents to distinguish compassionately between cultural stereotypes and biblical truth. Often, real men are portrayed as hairy, dirty construction workers who hunt and fish, while authentic women are portrayed as pretty, passive, perfumed tea-sippers in makeup and skirts. However, in reality, some women are assertive, enjoy sports, and excel at physical labor, like

Solomon's woman of noble character (Prov 31:10–31). Meanwhile, some men may be gifted artists like Bezalel and Oholiab (Exod 31) or enjoy cooking like Jacob (Gen 25:27–29). Neutral activities, hobbies, hair styles, colors, and clothes can be a good compromise to start. Parents must use discernment when deciding which battles matter, and they must apply extra grace during the early stages of the journey. Time and love are the two most important factors. Parents must dispense these to their gender-dysphoric child liberally, even when embarrassed or disappointed by their child. And remember, when it comes to things like name-changing and cross-dressing, sometimes the most loving word a parent can say to their child is no.

Finally, for parents whose children have already begun or even completed the transition process, there are two important principles to remember. First, no prodigal is beyond the reach of Christ (Luke 15:11–32). Thank God our Lord came to redeem the sick, because it is they, and not the healthy, who need the great physician the most (Mark 2:17). So never give up on your child, even your fully transitioned adult transgender child, because such were some of us, but we were washed (1 Cor 6:9–11). Never giving up means that, like the father of the Mark 9 child, you never stop praying for your child, never cut your child out of your life completely, and never affirm their decision to transition. This is a delicate balance, but one that must be maintained with compassion. Remember, you will never help your child if you act without love (1 Cor 13:1–3). And second, you need to get active. Others can benefit from your struggles, successes, mistakes, regrets, victories, and even failures. It is not enough to sit back and say, "Puberty-suppressing hormones are not my problem," while children are butchered and disfigured in the name of gender affirmation. Desistance can occur at any time in life, and adults who have sought chemical and even surgical transition have later repented and detransitioned.[3] As a parent, you need to know and exercise your rights (Acts 16:37). Gender affirmation proponents are engaged in unethical behavior and, in most cases, they do not even

3. Singal, "Your Child Says She's Trans," 98.

operate by their own radical policies and standards. Therefore, as a parent who has lost control of their child due to manipulation, legal battles, or age of majority, it is your responsibility to document every stage of their transition; note every objection; record the name of every doctor, therapist, counselor, or social worker; appeal every process; and do everything in your power to prevent your child from being coerced into making a painful, regrettable, irreversible decision. Any gender-affirming therapist who recommends puberty suppressors to a child that ultimately desists has misdiagnosed that child and is guilty of negligence. So is the doctor who prescribed the GnRH agonists, the activist who influenced the child, and everyone else involved with the transition process, including teachers, counselors, social workers, and media gurus. If at any point your child desists, then legal recourse can and should be pursued to the fullest extent of the law, and the negligent parties should be held fiscally, if not criminally, responsible. Misdiagnosing a child as transgender mars a human being for life and removes their ability to reproduce. If gender affirmation advocates are so confident that puberty-suppressing hormones are the proper course of treatment for all gender-dysphoric and TGNC children that they will legally bypass or override parental rights, then they should be held responsible for the pain and suffering that they directly or indirectly inflict if they are wrong. This may seem like a small consolation to a parent of a child whose gender dysphoria desists post-transition, but if enough misdiagnosed individuals sought civil and criminal justice, then future children may be spared from a lifetime of unnecessary suffering. As noted earlier, the most ethically suspect feature of the gender affirmation approach is that those who advocate for puberty-suppressing hormones are the ones who stand to benefit financially from the increased number of children pursuing this course of treatment.

Prescribing puberty-suppressing hormones to gender-dysphoric and TGNC children is a dangerous and unethical practice. It harms the child, overrides the parents' rights, constitutes an unjust distribution of benefits and burdens, ignores the distinction between male and female, and ultimately coerces a minor into permanently mutilating their body. So if you are the parent, the medical provider, or the ministry professional with a gender-dysphoric child in your life, and if, after you have examined the science, the studies, the Scriptures, and the ethics, you are convinced that this practice is unethical, then how will you respond to your child's request for GnRH agonists? Will you have the courage to say, "Little children, keep yourselves from puberty-suppressing hormones?" And what happens if they, or someone else in your life, one day asks you that one dreaded question: "Why?" Are you prepared to answer with gentleness and respect?

11

Why Shouldn't You Give Your Gender-dysphoric Child Puberty Suppressors?

YOU ARE THE PARENT, the medical care provider, or the ministry professional. There is a child in your family, your practice, or your church who is suffering from symptoms of gender dysphoria. After carefully considering the biological, etiological, and ethical elements of the gender affirmation approach, you are now in a position to help this child make a major decision that will affect them for the rest of their life. Can you, with a clear conscience, encourage this child to pursue puberty-suppressing hormones in order to treat their symptoms of gender dysphoria? For parents, medical practitioners, and ministry professionals who are seeking to help guide gender-dysphoric and TGNC children through a distressful period of adolescence, there are seven reasons to consider the gender affirmation approach of administering puberty-suppressing hormones as an unscientific, unethical, and medically unnecessary treatment option.

The first reason why puberty-suppressing hormones constitute unethical treatment of gender-dysphoric and TGNC children is because their very use is based on affirming the subjective self-diagnosis of a child who is unqualified to make a major medical diagnosis or decision. Contrary to the popular assertions of gender affirmation proponents, denying a child access to puberty-suppressing hormones neither ignores the child's state of distress nor subverts their autonomy. An appeal to autonomy does not mandate that minors receive unrestricted, long-term access to powerful, expensive, and unproven pharmaceuticals that will alter their body unnecessarily. Autonomy must be qualified by an understanding of the entire treatment process coupled with an absence of controlling influences. Not only do children and adolescents fail to meet both qualifications, but the principle of paternalism requires that parents, medical providers, and ministers serve as gatekeepers to unethical treatment options. Gender-affirmation advocates recognize as much in letter, but ignore these principles in practice. For example, WPATH's *Standards of Care* identifies the fourth minimum criteria for administering puberty-suppressing hormones as follows: "The adolescent has given informed consent and, particularly when the adolescent has not reached the age of consent, the parents or other caretakers or guardians have consented to the treatment."[1] Since adolescents are generally incapable of meeting the bioethical criteria for informed consent, and since gender affirmation advocates stand to benefit from the child's transition, any biochemical treatment of the child without parental consent or any attempt to coerce consent from the parents must be deemed an ethical violation of policy and procedure.

The second reason to reject the gender affirmation approach to treating gender dysphoria stems from the fact that medicine is not practiced in a moral vacuum. The administration of puberty-suppressing hormones violates the established framework of bioethical norms, particularly nonmaleficence. GnRH agonists, when prescribed to gender-dysphoric children, do pose the serious and permanent threat of harm to the physical, emotional, psychological, and spiritual development of the child. This harm, which interferes with the process of puberty, alters the child's brain, stunts the child's growth, prevents the child's fertility, and wreaks havoc on the child's endocrine system which contradicts the standard

1. Coleman et al., "Standards of Care," 19.

Hippocratic Oath of medicine, an oath that, while consistent with evangelical principles, predates New Testament Christianity. Furthermore, GnRH agonists do not resolve any distress that results from sexual trauma, autism, family dysfunction, sinful behavior, or any other environmental factors. Instead, puberty suppression will only serve to mask or aggravate these symptoms, thereby contributing to the child's distress. Even WPATH's *Standards of Care* identifies the third minimum criteria for administering puberty-suppressing hormones as follows: "Any co-existing psychological, medical, or social problems that could interfere with treatment . . . have been addressed."[2] However, in practice, gender affirmation therapists are diagnosing gender dysphoria and encouraging children to pursue puberty suppression without considering any of these elements. Therefore, failure to address all comorbid factors in a rush to administer puberty suppressors will not only harm the child, but also constitutes a serious ethical violation.

The third reason why puberty-suppressing hormones comprise an unethical practice is due to the fact that they have neither been scientifically tested nor officially approved for treating gender-dysphoric and TGNC children. Prescribing puberty-suppressing hormones in order to resolve the psychological distress of gender dysphoria in children remains an off-label use of a powerful and expensive synthetic pharmaceutical that was originally developed for the treatment of the physical condition of precocious puberty. The gender affirmation approach itself constitutes an experimental treatment of gender dysphoria, not evidence-based medicine. The trial-and-error mindset of gender affirmation is best illustrated by Dr. Ehrensaft's testimony recorded in the section evaluating gender affirmation. Hruz et al. explain the problem with the experimental nature of prescribing puberty-suppressing hormones as follows:

> Experimental medical treatments for children must be subject to especially intense scrutiny, since children cannot provide legal consent to medical treatment of any kind (parents or guardians must consent for their child to receive treatment), to say nothing of consenting to

2. Coleman et al., "Standards of Care," 19.

become research subjects for testing an unproven therapy. In the case of gender dysphoria, however, the safety
and efficacy of puberty-suppressing hormones is not well
founded in evidence . . . Whether puberty suppression
is safe and effective when used for gender dysphoria
remains unclear and unsupported by rigorous scientific
evidence.[3]

However, proponents of gender affirmation continue to disregard the impulsive nature of children and proceed to advocate for
puberty suppression at the first signs of gender dysphoria in spite
of their own guidelines recorded in WPATH's *Standards of Care*.
These guidelines identify the first minimum criteria for pursuing
synthetic puberty suppression as, "The adolescent has demonstrated a long-lasting and intense pattern of gender nonconformity or
gender dysphoria."[4] This brash experimentation on a generation of
children under the guise of evidence-based medicine constitutes a
violation of biomedical ethics.

Fourth, it is deliberately misleading to maintain that the
long-term use of puberty-suppressing hormones for the treatment
of gender dysphoria is either safe or void of permanent side effects.
Even though the presumptions of safety and reversibility have become a rallying cry for gender affirmation advocates who claim to
practice evidence-based medicine, no evidence exists to support
these claims. On the contrary, evidence is mounting to refute the
assertion that synthetic hormone treatment has been proven safe
and effective treatment for gender dysphoria. First, an increasing
number of medical professionals, including Cretella and Hruz et
al., have advised against this treatment option, outlining the dan-
gers of puberty suppression. Second, ethicists such as Abel, Dreger, and Drescher and Pula have advised caution by questioning
both the practices and the politics that guide the use of puberty
suppression. And finally, even WPATH's *Standards of Care* has
warned, "Neither puberty suppression nor allowing puberty to occur is a neutral act . . . there are concerns about negative physical

3. Hruz et al., "Growing Pains," 14–15.
4. Coleman et al., "Standards of Care," 19.

side effects of GnRH analogue use."[5] The only scientific evidence that gender affirmation advocates can appeal to in an attempt to support the claims of safety and reversibility is derived from the limited conclusions of GnRH agonist use to treat precocious puberty. As examined in the section of anatomy and physiology, this use of synthetic hormones on children with precocious puberty is a completely different condition for which GnRH agonists are medically necessary. The long-term effects of GnRH agonists on the hypothalamus and pituitary gland of gender-dysphoric children—the two main components of the endocrine system located in the brain—are completely unknown. Meanwhile, the effects of puberty suppressors on the reproductive system and bone development are known to be harmful and, therefore, unethical.

The fifth reason to consider puberty-suppressing hormones unethical results from the looping effect that the gender affirmation approach has on children.[6] Based on the plastic and elastic nature of gender identity that all but the most radical proponents of gender affirmation acknowledge, this method of treatment arguably manipulates children into a course of permanent medical action they would never otherwise pursue and will likely later regret. The phenomenon of neuroplasticity results in a self-fulfilling prophecy when gender-dysphoric children are exposed to gender affirmation methods over time. Evidence to support this assertion is derived from the fact that, in spite of the established 80 percent desistance rate, 100 percent of the children that were prescribed GnRH agonists in one test case persisted to cross-sex hormone therapy and ultimately pursued transition surgeries. Therefore, even WPATH's *Standards of Care* warns that GnRH agonists are not a neutral approach to buy time. Instead, they represent an active, unethical approach to treating gender-dysphoric and TGNC children that violates the autonomy of the patient by influencing the child to pursue life-altering medical treatment at an impressionable age that they would not have otherwise pursued (Rom 1:32).

5. Coleman et al., "Standards of Care," 20.
6. Hruz et al., "Standards of Care," 25.

The desistance rate, which is another piece of evidence that both proponents and critics of gender affirmation agree exists, is the sixth reason to consider puberty-suppressing hormones as unethical treatment for gender-dysphoric and TGNC children. With desistance rates recognized at 80 percent, four out of every five children who self-diagnose as gender dysphoric will eventually resolve their distress and identify with their natal gender. Radical members of the gender affirmation movement, such as Temple Newhook et al., have attempted to circumvent the desistance rate with statistical manipulation. This has resulted in gender affirmation colleagues such as Zucker, a contributing author to WPATH's *Standards of Care,* responding to these claims by declaring that even a persistence rate of 40 percent is absurd, lacking any evidence to substantiate the claim. The established desistance of the overwhelming majority of gender-dysphoric and TGNC children renders the use of puberty-suppressing hormones unnecessary, unjust, and unethical. Parents, medical practitioners, and ministry professionals alike should exercise the ethical practices of gatekeeping and paternalism and seek an alternative method of treatment in the best interest of the child.

And finally, the administration of puberty-suppressing hormones under the auspices of gender affirmation violates the biblical principles of gender and human sexuality. Scripture records that all human beings possess the image of God, expressed as either male or female (Gen 1:26–27). This creation account is reiterated by the New Testament teachings of Christ (Matt 19:4). Maleness and femaleness are neither socially constructed nor assigned at birth, but is an innate part of each human being from conception (Ps 139:13). Scientific analysis of human DNA affirms the unique maleness and femaleness of human beings, as Nicholi observes:

> Sexuality . . . contributes to our identity as living beings. We are either male or female—and we have little choice. Our genetic makeup, the particular combination of x and y chromosomes, determines our sexual identity. These genes and certain chemical substances called hormones—their relative presence or absence in the

body—determine how masculine or feminine we appear physically and the intensity of our sexual desire.[7]

No amount of social, chemical, or physical manipulation can alter the innate maleness or femaleness of a human being. Even a natal male who follows every aspect of gender affirmation protocol from birth through adulthood, including social transition, puberty suppression, cross-sex hormones, top surgery, and bottom surgery, will still possess XY chromosomes. The best modern medicine can provide under gender affirmation is a mutilated body and a strong delusion in an attempt to disguise the innate sexual nature that God endows to each human being at the moment of conception. For these seven reasons, the practice of prescribing puberty-suppressing hormones to gender-dysphoric and TGNC children is unethical.

7. Nicholi, "Human Sexuality," 341.

12

What Would You Say to a Child Who Really Wants Puberty Suppressors?

IF YOU ARE A child experiencing distress over your gender, then you are probably not too happy with me right now. And to be honest, I don't blame you. I just wrote a book explaining how something you want is wrong and dangerous and harmful and should be avoided at all costs. Who do I think I am to tell you how to feel or what to do, right?

Well, I am a pastor. And that means I attend at a lot of funerals. Sadly, I have lost count of how many funerals I have overseen where the deceased succumbed to a drug overdose. But I still remember the first one I ever conducted. It involved a young man that I never met in life. I never even met his family until after he died. They were calling around to churches to find someone who would say something at his funeral, and I agreed to speak for them.

On the day before the funeral, I drove over to his home to meet with his family. When I arrived, there were about twenty people crammed into a small living room, all of them waiting for me. His parents, his grandparents, his brothers and sisters, and even his two young children were there, and all of them were wishing he would walk through the door instead of me. Some of them wondered why he was not coming home. It was so sad.

I sat there and listened to them tell story after story of this young man's life, and it broke my heart. The young man was loved by his family, he had so much to offer, and he was going to be greatly missed! Those are the times when I wish I had magic words that would take the pain away, but those words do not exist. When they finished telling me about the young man's life, I asked them if there was anything I could do for them.

The young man's mom said, "Yes. There is one thing you can do." She went on to say, "We understand that all of his friends are planning to be at the funeral. And, as far as we know, many of them use drugs. This is why we called you. Promise me that you will tell them that the drugs they use are killing them too. Promise me you will tell them that, if they want to honor my son, then they should get clean, not high." I promised.

There was a really big crowd at the funeral the next day. This young man had so many friends, and they were all sad, angry, confused, and hurting. So when it was time to speak, even though part of me was dreading it, I stood up in front of this group of strangers and I began to talk about a man who everyone else in the room knew better than I did. I started by sharing a little bit about the things that were important to him, and that part was received well. Then I shared the gospel. I do not know if anyone trusted Christ to save them on that day or not, but they did listen politely. And finally, just before I closed, I honored his mother's request, and I shared the message she made me promise to deliver. I told them all, as gently as I could, that the same drugs that killed their friend would one day claim their lives if they did not get help and get clean. And even though I did not talk long or loud, I made a room full of people very angry. I knew they were angry because some of them stood up and stormed out as soon as I mentioned drugs. A few even approached me after the funeral and said some things to me that I will not repeat. Others would not even look at me after the funeral.

On that day of my first drug overdose funeral, and at every one since, I made a lot of people very angry, and I knew that was going to happen. I knew it, because I had to tell them something they did not want to hear. People who use drugs often do it because they really want to use them. Sometimes the feeling is so strong that they start to believe they cannot live without the drugs. They do not want to hear someone like me tell them drugs are bad. They want to hear that they are going to be fine. So, do you want to know why I told them what they did not want to hear, even though I knew it was going to make them mad? I said it because it was the right thing to do. The truth is always right, even when it is not what you want to hear. So I told them the truth. I would rather have them hate me for telling the hard truth than love me for telling a happy lie. A lie could kill them. But the truth would set them free. That is why I told them the truth. And that is why I wrote this book.

If you are like most children who are experiencing gender dysphoria, then you would probably much rather hear how puberty-suppressing hormones will make you happy, and how a transition to the opposite gender will ultimately solve all of your problems. But the truth is, it will not. Gender transition is a lie that will cause you great pain if you continue down that path. The truth is that, while it might not be easy or pleasant at first, you will be much happier by learning to accept the gender God gave you. You are not a mistake. You are fearfully and wonderfully made (Ps 139:14). And God knows you (Matt 10:29–31). And, best of all, God loves you (Eph 2:4)!

You might think, "How could God love me?" Listen, there are no perfect people in this world. We all sin and fall short of God's glory (Rom 3:23). And we all have our struggles. Some people struggle with drugs and alcohol. Others struggle with anger, honesty, gender, or sexuality. In the end, the bad news is that we all deserve to be punished by God for our sin (Rom 6:23). The good news is that God has provided a way to save us (Rom 5:8). Jesus Christ, the Son of God, became one of us (Rom 5:8). He lived a perfect life in our place, died a sacrificial death on the cross for our sins, and then rose from the dead (John 3:16). So if you acknowledge that Jesus is Lord, and that his sacrifice paid for your sins, then you will be saved (Rom 10:9). You do not have to do anything to be forgiven, only believe (Eph 2:8–9).

The even better news is that salvation is not where your relationship with Christ ends. It is just the beginning. Once you are saved, God desires to change you (Eph 2:10). This includes some big changes about the way you think about yourself as male or female (Rom 12:1–2). Now, change is not always easy or pleasant, but with Christ, change is possible (1 John 4:4).

If you are a child struggling with your gender identity, then you are standing at a major fork on the road of your life. On the one hand, if you choose the gender affirmation path, you are going to begin taking dangerous, expensive, and experimental medication for a long time. Some people will try to convince you that the effects of this medication are tested, safe, and reversible. But as I explained in this book, they are not. The truth is that this medication will not turn you into the opposite gender, but it will keep you from developing the way God designed you. Over time, you will have to take even more chemicals. These chemicals will be even more painful and destructive, they will cause damage to your body, and the results will not be reversible. Finally, you will begin a lifetime process of surgeries in an attempt to disguise your natal gender. These surgeries will be complicated, painful, and expensive, and they will leave you disappointed and unable to have children of your own one day. One the other hand, if you choose the path of accepting your natal gender, your first few steps will be difficult. This is the truth, too. It is never easy to walk in one direction when your feelings or your heart are trying to pull you in another one. But if you follow the guidelines I laid out in this book, surround yourself with loving family and good friends, and walk with the Lord, then you will find peace. I hope, by having your parent, doctor, or pastor read this book, and by having you read this chapter, you choose to let God change your heart rather than letting men and women alter your body. I know this may not be what you wanted to hear, but it is true. May God bless you and guide you in all truth.

Bibliography

Abel, Brendan S. "Hormone Treatment of Children and Adolescents With Gender Dysphoria: An Ethical Analysis." *The Hastings Center Report,* (Sept/Oct 2014) 23–27.

Beauchamp, Tom L., and James F. Childress. *Principles of Biomedical Ethics.* 7th ed. New York: Oxford University Press, 2013.

Calfas, Jennifer. "An Ohio Bill Would Force Teachers and Doctors to Out Transgender Children." http://time.com/5330293/ohio-bill-transgender-youth/.

Cohen-Kettenis, Peggy T., et al. "Puberty Suppression in a Gender-dysphoric Adolescent: A 22-Year Follow-Up." *Archives of Sexual Behavior* 40 (Aug 2011) 843–47.

Coleman, E., et al. "Standards of Care for the Health of Transsexual, Transgender, and Gender-nonconforming People, Version 7," *International Journal of Transgenderism* 13 (2012) 1–112.

Compton, Julie. "'Boy or Girl?' Parents Raising 'Theybies' Let Kids Decide." https://www.nbcnews.com/feature/nbc-out/boy-or-girl-parents-raising-theybies-let-kids-decide-n891836.

Cretella, Michelle. "Gender Dysphoria in Children: American College of Pediatricians." *Issues in Law & Medicine* 32 (Fall 2017) 287–304.

———. "Gender Dysphoria in Children and Suppression of Debate." *Journal of American Physicians and Surgeons* 21 (Summer 2016) 50–54.

Dean, Jamie. "Suffer the Children." https://world.wng.org/2017/03/suffer_the_children.

Dellaperute, Michael. "The Church and the Transgender Issue." *The Journal of Ministry and Theology* 20 (Spring 2016) 76–122.

de S. Cameron, Nigel M. "Bioethics: The Twilight of Christian Hippocratism." In *God and Culture* D. A. Carson and John D. Woodbridge, 321–40. Grand Rapids: Eerdmans, 1993.

de Vries, Annelou, et al. "Autism Spectrum Disorders in Gender-dysphoric Children and Adolescents." *Journal of Autism & Developmental Disorders* 40 (Aug 2010) 930–36.

Dreger, Alice. "Gender Identity Disorder in Childhood: Inconclusive Advice to Parents." *The Hastings Center Report* (Jan/Feb 2009) 26–29.

Dresher, Jack, and Jack Pula. "Ethical Issues Raised by the Treatment of Gendervariant Prepubescent Children." *The Hastings Center Report* (Sept/Oct 2014) 17–22.

Firth, Malcom. "Childhood Abuse and Depressive Vulnerability in Clients With Gender Dysphoria." *Counseling and Psychotherapy Research* 14 (Dec 2014) 297–305.

Fox, Fallon. "Leelah Alcorn's Suicide: Conversion Therapy is Child Abuse." http://time.com/3655718/leelah-alcorn-suicide-transgender-therapy/.

Geisler, Norman. *Christian Ethics: Opinions and Issues.* Grand Rapids: Baker, 1999.

Giovanardi, Guido. "Buying Time or Arresting Development? The Dilemma of Administering Hormone Blockers in Trans Children and Adolescents." *Porto Biomedical Journal* 2 (Sept/Oct 2017) 153–56.

Hann, Miranda, et al. "Bioethics in Practice: Ethical Issues in the Care of Transgender Patients." *The Ochsner Journal* 17 (Summer 2017) 144–45.

Harris, Mary. "I'd Rather Have a Living Son than a Dead Daughter." August 2, 2016. Radio interview. 28:32. https://www.wnycstudios.org/story/id-rather-have-living-son-dead-daughter/.

Hruz, Paul, et al. "Growing Pains: Problems With Puberty Suppression in Treating Gender Dysphoria." *New Atlantis* 52 (Spring 2017) 3–36.

Johnson, Jon. "What is the Function of the Hypothalamus?" https://www.medicalnewstoday.com/articles/312628.php.

Kuper, Laura. "Puberty Blocking Medications: Clinical Research Review." http://impactprogram.org/wp-content/uploads/2014/12/Kuper-2014-Puberty-Blockers-Clinical-Research-Review.pdf.

Kuvalanka, Katherine A., et al. "Trans and Gender-nonconforming Children and Their Caregivers: Gender Presentations, Peer Relations, and Well-Being at Baseline." *Journal of Family Psychology* 31 (June 2017) 889–99.

Littman, Lisa. "Rapid-onset Gender Dysphoria in Adolescents and Young Adults: A Study of Parental Reports." *PLoS ONE* 13 (2018) 1–41.

Martini, Fredric H., et al. *Visual Anatomy and Physiology.* 2nd ed. Boston: Pearson, 2015.

McQuilkin, Robertson, and Paul Copan. *An Introduction to Biblical Ethics.* 3rd ed. Downers Grove, IL: Intervarsity, 2014.

Meier, Colt, and Julie Harris. "Fact Sheet: Gender Diversity and Transgender Identity in Children." http://www.apadivisions.org/division-44/resources/advocacy/transgender-children.pdf.

Nicholi, Armand, Jr. "Human Sexuality: A Psychiatric and Biblical Perspective." In *God and Culture*, edited by D. A. Carson and John D. Woodbridge, 341–55. Grand Rapids: Eerdmans, 1993.

Puckett, Jae A., et al. "Barriers to Gender-affirming Care for Transgender and Gender Non-conforming Individuals." *Sexuality Research & Social Policy* 15 (Mar 2018) 48–59.

Ristori, Jiska, and Thomas D. Steensma. "Gender Dysphoria in Childhood." *International Review of Psychiatry* 28 (2016) 13–20.

Sieczkowski, Cavan. "Mom's Birth Announcement for Transgender Son is Something to Celebrate." https://www.huffingtonpost.com/2014/12/02/mom-birth-announcement-transgender-son_n_6254446.html.

Sifferlin, Alexandra. "Gender Confirmation Surgery is on the Rise in the U.S." http://time.com/4787914/transgender-gender-confirmation-surgery/.

Singal, Jesse. "Your Child Says She's Trans. She Wants Hormones and Surgery. She's 13." *The Atlantic* 322 (Jul/Aug 2018) 88–107.

Stevens, Jaime, et al. "Insurance Coverage of Puberty Blocker Therapies for Transgender Youth." *Pediatrics* 136 (Dec 2015) 1029–31.

Temple Newhook, Julia, et al. "A Critical Commentary on Follow-up Studies and 'Desistance' Theories about Transgender and Gender-nonconforming Children." *International Journal of Transgenderism* 19 (Apr/June 2018) 212–24.

Walker, Andrew T. *God and the Transgender Debate*. Purcellville, VA: The Good Book, 2018.

Ward, Susan L., et al. *Maternal-Child Nursing Care*. Philadelphia: F. A. Davis, 2016.

Wesson, Kenneth. "A Primer on Neuroplasticity: Experience and Your Brain." https://brainworldmagazine.com/a-primer-on-neuroplasticity-experience-and-your-brain/.

Winters, Kelley, et al. "Learning to Listen to Trans and Gender Diverse Children: A Response to Zucker (2018) and Steensa and Cohen-Kettenis (2018)," *International Journal of Transgenderism* 19 (Apr/June 2018) 246–50.

Yarhouse, Mark. *Understanding Gender Dysphoria*. Downers Grove, IL: IVP, 2015.

Zucker, Kenneth. "The Myth of Persistence: Response to 'A Critical Commentary on Follow-up Studies and "Desistance" Theories about Transgender and Gender Non-conforming Children' by Temple Newhook et al." *International Journal of Transgenderism* 19 (Apr/June 2018) 231–45.

Index

Abel, Brendan
  autonomy as support for
    hormone treatments, 67
  criteria for autonomy in
    children, 68
  discontinuing suppression
    therapy, 42–43
  effects of GnRH agonists, 64
  ethical considerations of puberty
    suppression, 12
  failure to accommodate effects
    on behavior, 49
  gender affirmation appeals to
    beneficence, 71
  obligation to help patients, 69
Accommodation model, 46. *See
  also* Gender affirmation
  approach
Adolescents
  cognitive immaturity of, 68–69
  criteria for administering
    puberty-suppression
    hormones, 86
  criteria for autonomy in, 84
  GnRH agonists effects on, 27
  persistence and desistance in, 40
  rapid onset of dysphoria in, 12
  therapeutic model treatment
    in, 55
  treatment decisions for, 68–69
Adrenal gland maturation, 22

Affirmation of child, 4
Affirmation process. *See* Gender
  affirmation approach
Affirming care. *See* Gender
  affirmation approach
Alcorn, Leelah, 54
American Psychiatric Association
  Task Force on the Treatment
  of Gender Identity, 45
Anatomic dysphoria, 11
Anatomic sex, 27
Androgen Insensitivity Syndrome
  (AIS), 36
Androgens
  production during puberty, 20
  in progression of puberty, 22
Assigned sex. *See* Natal gender
Autism Spectrum Disorder (ASD)
  as comorbid factor in dysphoria,
    70, 79
  with gender dysphoria, 35
  GnRH agonists effects on, 85
Autonomic functions, 19
Autonomy, principle of
  children's right to, 49, 67
  criteria for children, 68–69,
    84, 87
  defined, 62–63
  ethical respect for, 61
  factors in modification of, 62–63

99